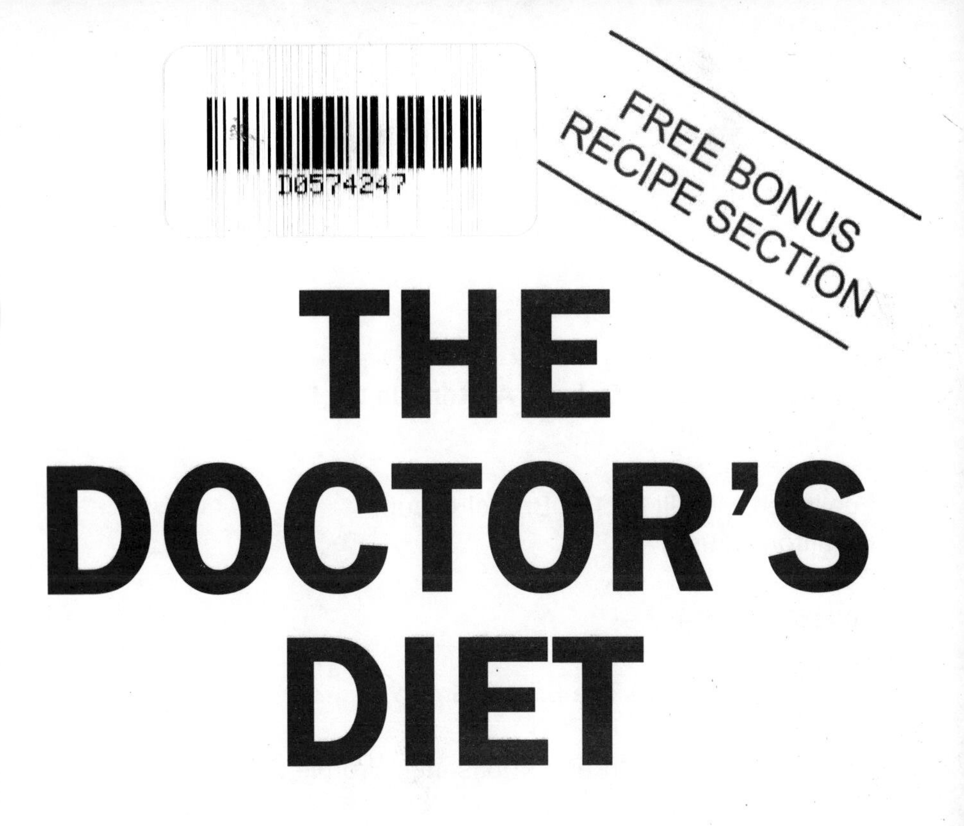

THE DOCTOR'S DIET

To Lose A Stone In 10 Days

Dr Michael Spira

The Doctor's Diet: To Lose A Stone In 10 Days
Dr Michael Spira

Published MMVIII by The Bristol Group,
Hamilton House,
2 Station Road,
Epping CM16 4HA

Typeset by SJ Design and Publishing, Bromley, Kent

ISBN 1-903904-72-2

Contents

About the author:

Dr Michael Spira was for over 30 years senior partner in a UK group practice with a special interest in Diabetes and Obesity. During the same period he was Consulting Physician to BUPA Wellness, London, where he counselled literally thousands of clients (including many 'celebs') on lifestyle and diet. For many years he was Medical Consultant both to the UK's second largest group of slimming clubs and to one of the UK's leading slimming magazines. He has broadcast many times on national TV and radio and he has written several books on diet and nutrition.

Chapter 1

Why This Book?

As there are so many diet books you may well ask, "Why another book?". Before I answer that I'll let you into a secret. For some time now I have been promising myself I would never write another diet book. Over the years I've written three including the bestselling *How To Lose Weight Without Really Dieting.* I felt that that book said everything worthwhile knowing about a healthy way to lose and maintain weight. It was based on a low fat approach and, when originally published, was well ahead of the game. Nowadays, of course, low fat is all the rage, along with high fats/low carbs.

So, I said to myself, I knew all there was to know about diets and I had written it all down. Right?

Wrong.

So what happened? The best way for me to explain is to talk about one of my patients. John is a 55 year old top executive who came to se me at my Wellness clinic in London. I arranged for him to have an EBCT heart scan. The scanner shoots out electron beams at the heart to take special pictures of the coronary arteries. The machine can tell how much calcium there is in the arteries – the more calcium the more likely that CHD (coronary heart disease) is present. We were both shocked to find that he had a medium calcium score – certainly more than he should have had for a healthy man of his age. The result came as a complete surprise because, apart from slightly raised blood pressure, he had none of the risk factors for CHD such as smoking, diabetes, too much alcohol, high cholesterol, family history. Our only slight concern was that, although he wasn't really overweight, he had a little too much 'tummy' – he'd been buying trousers with a slightly larger waist over the past few years!

I arranged for John to have a nuclear heart scan which shows how well the heart is perfused with blood. The higher the perfusion the less significant CHD is present. Whilst John was waiting for the result of the scan he pondered the wisdom of having started down this route. After all, he hadn't had any symptoms of CHD. Why was he giving himself all this hassle?

The radiologist in charge of the scan came to see him. "Do you want the good news or the bad first?" she asked. "Hit me with either," John said. "The bad news is that we've wasted your time because the good news is that your scan is perfectly normal."

Phew! A waste of time? Definitely not. Because of this 'scare' John had reached the end of this journey a much wiser man with knowledge that would probably save his life. You see, immediately after John's EBCT scan, I explained to John the importance of diet. And it is this knowledge that I want to share with you in this book.

I started by telling John about a friend of mine who is also a doctor. I explained that this doctor, when he was in his early 30s, was overweight and well on the road to becoming a type 2 diabetic – that's someone whose diabetes is generally controlled by diet, either alone or in combination with tablets. He then discovered that he was eating all the wrong foods. By changing his diet he stopped his condition progressing to diabetes and he lost considerable weight.

Let me repeat that last sentence. By *changing* his diet – NOT *going on* a diet – he stopped his condition progressing to diabetes *and he lost considerable weight.*

I then explained how type 2 diabetes and CHD are simply two different aspects of the same condition – variously known as the Metabolic Syndrome or Syndrome X. By changing his diet, not only did the doctor lose weight and prevent diabetes, he also drastically reduced his risk of developing CHD.

This was all music to John's ears. After all, what sane person wouldn't jump at the opportunity to:

1. Lose weight without going on a diet that made him or her go hungry?
2. Reduce the risk of developing diabetes?
3. Reduce the risk of developing CHD?

Remember, this was at a time when high fat low carbohydrate diets were all the rage in spite of all their health risks.

John followed my guidelines. And within two weeks he had lost 8lb and an inch from his waistline – without going hungry, without feeling faint or dizzy, without feeling nausea: in fact, without any of the side-effects often associated with many popular diets. In fact, he never felt better. He had more energy and more drive. And when I rechecked his cholesterol and blood sugar after a few weeks they were even better than before.

To say he was thrilled would be an understatement. He asked me to tell him of a book that he could recommend to his friends. Now, although there are several books around that tell a similar story, none of them do it in a way which all the people I knew who wanted to follow the diet found particularly helpful. Some books concentrated purely on the health benefits, especially for diabetes or heart disease, whereas others were full of recipes whose ingredients were not always easy to find. I wanted a book that would:

1. Explain the diet in simple terms;
2. Show how the diet would help people lose weight easily, painlessly *and healthily* as well as provide health benefits;
3. Have easy-to-prepare tasty recipes with easy-to-find ingredients.

Because I couldn't find such a book I did the obvious: I decided to write my own book. After all, I had written diet books before as well as publishing hundreds of articles in national magazines and being slimming adviser to two leading UK nationwide slimming organisations.

BUT WHAT IS SO SPECIAL ABOUT *THIS* BOOK?

To answer that let's look at what is currently around. There are two diets which are popular. The low fat diets, such as Weightwatchers, certainly cut down the calories but fail to address the problem of the wrong kind of carbs. The other popular diet, the high protein, high fat, low carbohydrate diet, such as Atkins, quite rightly is concerned with carbs, so much so that carbs as a group of nutrients are virtually banned. Quite apart from the unpalatability of such a diet there are serious potential health problems.

We'll look at these and other diets in more detail in Chapter 2. For now, it's important to stress that a good diet for weight loss and weight maintenance is a lifelong issue. This is where the diet I describe in my book scores. It doesn't cause side-effects. People feel well on it from Day One, and they and their families can follow the diet for the rest of their lives because they feel so good on it, they can eat food they enjoy, and they don't feel hungry. Then there is the added bonus that such a diet will also reduce the risk of heart disease and diabetes.

This book is not so much a diet, more a way of eating.

Chapter 2

Other Popular Diets – What's Wrong With Them?

Let's look at some of the most popular diets currently.

LOW FAT DIETS (EG WEIGHTWATCHERS)

These have been around for several years and are the diets used by many nationwide slimming clubs both in the UK and USA. They are based on the fact that fats in your diet are what is known as 'calorie-dense'. This means that they provide more calories, about 7 calories a gram, compared with carbohydrates and protein which each contain just 4 calories a gram. Which means, in theory at least, that you can eat almost twice as much carbohydrate or protein as you can fat and still put on only the same amount of weight. Or, to put it another way, for each gram of fat you cut out of your diet you will lose almost twice as much weight as you would for each gram of carbohydrate or protein.

So everyone who goes on a low fat diet loses weight. Yes? Of course not. Some will lose weight, but a lot will fail. Why? Because the calorie density of fat, carbohydrate and protein is only *part* of the story. What low fat diet enthusiasts fail to understand is that carbohydrates are just as important in what they do for your weight because of the way your body handles them. We'll look at that in the next chapter.

So if carbohydrates are so important, perhaps we should cut them out. Well, that's certainly the thinking behind the other most popular diets…

HIGH PROTEIN, HIGH FAT, LOW CARBOHYDRATE DIETS (EG ATKINS)

Quite rightly, these diets recognise the important part that carbohydrates can play in preventing weight loss. And there is no question that lots of people lose lots of weight on these diets, at least to begin with. Recent research in the USA which followed up slimmers on high protein/fat, low carbohydrate diets found that, whilst there was dramatic weight loss to begin with, after 12 months the weight loss was no greater than on a low fat diet.

So what's so wrong with these diets? One mistake is that they allow – indeed, encourage – any and all dietary fats. We'll see later in this book how dangerous that can be. But an even bigger mistake they make is that they treat *all* carbohydrates as villains. This just isn't so. Research over the past few years has shown that different carbohydrates have completely different effects on our bodies with completely different consequences for our weight. Some carbohydrates, especially most fruit and some vegetables banned by these diets, not only have little effect on weight loss but they also provide essential vitamins and antioxidants without which serious health problems may arise – not straightaway but gradually with time. These include an increased risk of coronary heart disease, stroke, kidney disease, breast cancer and osteoporosis. Not to mention of course that many people feel unwell on these diets. And besides, how many of us want to go without bread and potatoes for the rest of our lives?

OTHER DIETS

There are so many other diets. Some are based on eating a single food, such as cabbage soup. Quite apart from the serious lack of nutrients, how boring is that? Others base your food on your blood type. Sorry, but there's no science behind that. Another popular diet is food combining. Typically you avoid eating protein and carbohydrate at the same meal. Again, no science behind that. If it works, and sometimes it does, it is because you are watching what you eat and cutting back your calories which of course will result in weight loss.

The list of diets, many of them cranky, is almost endless. If they work – if you lose weight on them – it's always at a price. Either they don't provide all-important vitamins and antioxidants or they make you feel ill or they make you go hungry. A good diet for weight loss and weight maintenance is a lifelong issue. It is part of what should be a healthy lifestyle. It should be a way of eating that suits the whole family. A good diet is important right from early childhood. If we give our children the wrong kinds of food we are storing up health problems for them in the future.

There is only one diet that:

- ❑ works *and*

- ❑ helps you lose weight *and*
- ❑ doesn't make you go hungry *and*
- ❑ allows you to eat most of your favourite foods *and*
- ❑ not only doesn't make you feel ill but actually makes you feel well *and*
- ❑ not only does it not put you at risk of health problems it actually cuts your health risks.

Lots of *'ands'* – but that's why it's such a good diet. So read on.

But first, what about those carbs?

Chapter 3

Smart Carbs, Unsmart Carbs

"ALL CARBS ARE GOOD." "ALL CARBS ARE BAD."

Which is right? Your answer will depend on whom you believe. If you are a fan of low fat diets, such as Weightwatchers, you believe that it is only fats in your diet that matter and that the carbohydrates – or 'carbs' – are completely unimportant. Watch your fat intake and the carbs will take care of themselves.

But if you are a fan of high protein low carbohydrate diets, such as Atkins, the message you will have received loud and clear is that, providing you virtually eliminate all carbohydrates, the fats are completely unimportant. Eat as much artery-clogging fat as you like – you will still lose weight.

So where does the truth lie? The answer, as we saw in the previous chapter, is with neither. Time for a *short* lesson in nutrition and biology.

Our bodies need three sources of fuel: fats, carbs and proteins. Carbs are the fuels the body prefers as a source of glucose energy. Protein is converted to glucose if carbs aren't available. What about fat? This is the emergency fuel which is stored in case we starve. When food enters the stomach special chemicals called enzymes break it down so that the fats, carbs and proteins are absorbed into the bloodstream as small molecules. In the case of carbs these molecules are glucose.

Let's look at what happens to carbs, or glucose, next. They meet a hormone – insulin. The job of insulin, which is secreted by the pancreas gland, is to push glucose into our cells where it is converted to energy or stored as a larger chemical called glycogen. But that is not all that insulin does. One of its other important actions is to store fat.

So when we eat carbs the resultant glucose causes the release of insulin. The more glucose in our blood the more insulin we produce. And the more insulin we produce the more fat gets stored in our bodies – in other words, the fatter we get. And if we keep pushing insulin too much eventually insulin can't do its job of converting glucose to energy properly so that we have to produce more of it to do the job. This is called glucose intolerance. Our cells become resistant to insulin which is why we then need higher and higher levels. The result? High levels of insulin put down more and more fat in our bodies, so we put on weight. Eventually insulin resistance reaches a level when we become diabetic. That is what a particular kind of diabetes, know as type 2 diabetes, is – insulin resistance. Or, if it doesn't result in diabetes, it can cause a condition known as the Metabolic Syndrome or Syndrome X. This is a group of clinical features that includes high blood pressure, abdominal obesity (too much fat around the waist – the most dangerous place to store fat in terms of heart disease), glucose intolerance, and abnormal levels of blood fats (high triglycerides and low HDL or 'good' cholesterol).

Now up to this point fans of low carb diets have got it right. But from this point on they are completely wrong. You see, every carb is digested and absorbed at a different rate with different effects on blood levels of glucose. For example, white bread causes a rapid rise in blood glucose, whilst an apple causes a much lower rise. And of course the quicker the rise and the higher the level of blood glucose the more insulin is produced. And the more rapid and higher the rise the more rapid the subsequent fall in blood glucose.

Most of us have experienced the feeling of fullness immediately after eating a Chinese meal followed by hunger only two hours later. Why is this? Simply, the carbs in a Chinese meal, especially the white rice, cause rapid high levels of blood sugar, which satisfies hunger, followed by rapid falls, which makes us feel hungry again.

But look at what happens when we eat a meal that starts off perhaps with a small portion of pasta cooked *al dente*, followed by a main course of your favourite meat or fish with new potatoes and lots of green vegetables, followed by fruit salad (and, go on, have some custard too, if you like!). The *amount* of carbs may be the same, perhaps even higher, than in the Chinese meal. But the resulting blood glucose levels are much lower. Why? Because these kinds of carbs are digested and absorbed much more slowly. So we feel satisfied and we don't feel ravenous again two hours later. Just as important, our insulin levels haven't been pushed sky high.

So all carbs are different. Some cause rapid rises in blood glucose, others only gentle rises. The rate at which a particular carb causes blood glucose to rise is called its Glycaemic Index, or GI for short. A carb with a low GI causes gentle blood glucose rises, whereas a carb with a high GI causes steep rises. And of course this means that low GI carbs cause only gentle insulin production whilst high GI carbs cause high insulin production. Chapter 19 has a list of many common carbs divided into low, medium and high GI.

Incidentally, if you ever knew it, forget all that nonsense about 'complex carbohydrates', such as potatoes, being better for your blood glucose than 'simple carbohydrates'. That was based on pseudo-science which has been completely disproved. The chemical structure of a carb is no pointer to what it does to your blood glucose. The only way to find out, and the way researchers have discovered the GI values of carbs, is by laboriously feeding volunteers different carbs and then measuring their blood glucose responses over a period of several hours. That is why GI values are not yet available for all foods. But we have enough information to work out a really healthy and effective weight loss diet.

Why is the GI value different for different carbs? To answer that we need to look at what exactly a carb is. The simplest carb is a monosaccharide ('mono' meaning one, 'saccharide' meaning sweet). The most common monosaccharide is glucose. If two monosaccharides are joined together we have a disaccharide ('di' meaning two), the commonest example being sucrose or what we all know as table sugar. If lots of monosaccharides are joined together we get polysaccharides ('poly' meaning many), and these are known as starches which, unlike monosaccharides and disaccharides, are not sweet. Two common starches are amylose and amylopectin, the importance of which we'll see in a moment.

Another group of carbohydrates made up of lots of different monosaccharides are dietary fibres. The main difference between fibres and other carbs, such as sugar and starches, is that they are not broken down by the body's digestive system, so that they arrive at the large bowel unchanged.

Now we can look at why different carbs have different GI values.

1. The less a starch swells up when it is cooked (the technical term for which is 'gelatinised') the more slowly it is digested, and so the lower the GI. Examples of less starch gelatinisation, and so low GI, are long grain rice, brown rice and *al dente* spaghetti. More gelatinisation, and so higher GI, is seen in sticky white rice and overcooked pasta.
2. The more fibrous a food is the slower its digestion. This is because the fibrous coat around seeds and plant cells provides a physical barrier. Examples of fibrous food are whole-grain bread, Pumpernickel, lentils, All-Bran and barley, all of which have a low GI. Low fibre foods, with a high GI, include cornflakes and bagels.

3. The more amylose a food has compared with amylopectin the less the starch swells and the slower it is digested. Foods with a high amylose to amylopectin content, and therefore a low GI, include basmati rise, sweet potatoes and small new potatoes, whereas foods with a high amylopectin content and high GI include white rice and potatoes (other than small new ones).
4. The less processed a food is the larger the size of its particles and the more difficult it is for water and digestive enzymes to penetrate the higher surface area of the particles. This results in lower GI values as seen in stoneground whole-wheat bread and rolled oats. Highly processed foods with a high GI include instant oatmeal, rice cakes, and white bread.
5. Acidic foods slow down stomach emptying which slows down the rate at which starch is digested. Good examples are bread and pudding made from sourdough.
6. Surprisingly, the digestion of sugar produces far fewer glucose molecules than does the digestion of starch. For this reason some breakfast cereals and some biscuits that are quite high in sugar actually have fairly low GI values.
7. Fat also slows down stomach emptying and so slows down the digestion of starch. This is the reason that potato crisps have a lower GI than boiled or baked potatoes.

As I said earlier, the GI values of food cannot be predicted. They have to be worked out by measuring blood glucose levels after each food has been eaten. This has to be done on a large number of volunteers and on different samples of the same food type. This is the reason you will find variations in published GI values of foods. Also, the way a food is cooked will affect its GI value. Overcooked pasta has a much higher GI than that which is *al dente.*

Rice is another food whose GI varies according to its variety. This is because different rices contain different amounts of the starch, amylose. Amylose is digested slowly and the more that is present the lower the GI. Here are some typical GI values:

Parboiled rice	(During parboiling water-soluble nutrients pass from the outer layers to the inner, which makes this rice very nutritious)	44

Uncle Ben's Converted rice	(As parboiled rice)	44
Short grain Japanese rice	(Surprisingly low GI value which probably contributes to low prevalence of coronary heart disease in Japan)	48
Brown rice	(Long or medium grain nutty-flavoured rice – the most nutritious rice)	55
Long grain white rice	(Providing it isn't overcooked the rice grains remain separate)	56
Basmati rice	(Its lower GI value is due to its high amylose content)	58
Instant rice	(Commercially pre-cooked in order to shorten preparation time in the home)	87
Dessert rice	(High GI is due to absence of amylose)	88

For a classification of some common foods by their GI values go to Chapter 19.

Below is a table of GI values of some common foods. Don't treat the figures as gospel. There are enormous variations in samples of food depending on where it is grown or processed, how ripe it is (in the case of fruit), and how well cooked it is. Different researchers have found quite a variety of values for what would seem to be identical foods. This is why you may find different values for the same food in different books. As I have said earlier, working out the GI values of foods is not an exact science and there are all sorts of factors that can cause wide variations. So treat these figures as a rough guideline only.

First, here is a simple guide to the significance of a food's GI value:

GI less than 40: *very low GI*
GI 40-55: *low GI*
GI 55-70: *medium GI*
GI more than 70: *high GI*

BREADS & BAKERY

Bagel, white	72
Baguette, white, plain	95
Fruit loaf	44
Hamburger bun	61

Melba toast	70
Pumpernickel	50
Wholemeal rye bread	58
Rye bread	65
Sourdough rye	53
White flour bread	70
Wholemeal wheat flour (whole wheat) bread	71
Wholemeal flour	52
Multigrain	49
100% Whole Grain bread	51
Pita bread, white	57
Muffins, blueberry	59
BISCUITS	
Digestives	59
Oatcakes	57
Rich Tea	55
Shortbread	64
CRACKERS	
Cream Crackers	65
Puffed rice cakes, white	78
Rye crispbread	64
Water cracker	71
Wheat crackers	67
BREAKFAST CEREALS & RELATED PRODUCTS	
All-Bran	42
Bran Flakes	74
Coco Pops	77
Cornflakes	81
Frosties	55
Muesli	49
Oat bran, raw	55
Porridge made from rolled oats	58
Porridge, instant	66
Puffed Wheat	74
Rice Krispies	82
Shredded Wheat	75
Special K	69
Sultana Bran	73

Weetabix	70
Sweet corn	53
Couscous	65
Rice, white, boiled	64
Long grain, boiled	56
Basmati, white, boiled	58
Rice, brown	55
Instant rice, white, boiled	69
Parboiled rice	60
Converted, white, Uncle Ben's	42
Long grain, boiled	48
DAIRY PRODUCTS & ALTERNATIVES	
Custard	38
Ice cream, regular	61
Ice cream, low fat	43
Milk, full-fat	27
Milk, skimmed	32
Milk, condensed, sweetened	61
Yoghurt	
Yoghurt, regular	36
Yoghurt, fruit, low fat	26
Soy-based milk	
Soy milk, full fat	40
Soy milk, reduced fat	44
FRUIT AND FRUIT PRODUCTS	
Apples, raw	38
Apple juice, unsweetened	40
Apricots, raw	57
Apricots, tinned	64
Apricots, dried	31
Banana, raw	52
Cherries, raw	22
Dates, dried	103
Figs, dried	61
Grapefruit, raw	25
Grapefruit juice, unsweetened	48
Grapes, raw	46
Kiwi fruit, raw	53

Lychee, tinned	79
Mango, raw	51
Marmalade, orange	48
Oranges, raw	42
Orange juice	52
Pawpaw/papaya, raw	59
Peaches, raw	42
Peaches, tinned	38
Peach, tinned in natural juice	45
Pears, raw	38
Pears, tinned in natural juice	43
Pineapple, raw	59
Pineapple juice, unsweetened	46
Plums, raw	39
Prunes, pitted	29
Raisins	64
Strawberries, fresh	40
Strawberry jam	51
Sultanas	56
Tomato juice, unsweetened	38
Watermelon, raw	72
LEGUMES AND NUTS	
Baked Beans, tinned	40
Beans, dried, boiled	29
Butter Beans	31
Haricot beans	38
Kidney Beans	28
Lentils	26
Soya beans	18
MIXED MEALS & CONVENIENCE FOODS	
Chicken nuggets	46
Fish Fingers	38
Pizza, cheese	60
Pizza, vegetarian, thin and crispy	49
WHITE BREAD WITH SPREADS	
White bread with butter	59
White bread with skimmed milk cheese	55
White bread with butter and skim milk cheese	62

White/wholemeal wheat bread with peanut butter	59
PASTA and NOODLES	
Fettucine, egg	40
Gluten-free	54
Gnocchi	68
Instant noodles	48
Linguine, thick, durum wheat	46
Linguine, thin, durum wheat	52
Macaroni	47
Ravioli, durum wheat flour, meat filled	39
Rice noodles, dried, boiled	61
Rice noodles, freshly made, boiled	40
Spaghetti, white, boiled 5 min	38
Spaghetti, white, boiled 10 min	42
Spaghetti, white, boiled 20 min	61
Spaghetti, wholemeal, boiled	32
Vermicelli, white, boiled	35
SNACK FOODS AND CONFECTIONERY	
Chocolate, milk, plain	43
Corn chips	63
Jelly beans	78
Mars Bar	65
Muesli bar containing dried fruit	61
Cashew nuts, salted	22
Peanuts	14
Popcorn, plain	72
Potato crisps, plain, salted	54
Honey	55
VEGETABLES	
Green peas	48
Sweet corn	54
Beetroot	64
Carrots	47
Parsnips	97
Potato, baked	85
Potato, boiled	50
Potato, french fries	75
Potato, instant mashed	85

Potato, mashed	74
Potato, new	57
Sweet potato	61
Swede	72
Yam	37
ETHNIC	
Chapatti	58
Hummus	6
Stuffed grapevine leaves (rice and lamb stuffing with tomato sauce)	30
Glutinous rice	92
Jasmine rice	109
Lychee, canned in syrup	79
Rice cracker, plain	91
Rice noodles, dried, boiled	61
Rice noodles, fresh, boiled	40
Rice vermicelli	58
BEVERAGES	
Coca Cola	58
Lucozade	95
Juices	
Apple juice	40
Grapefruit juice, unsweetened	40
Orange juice	48
Pineapple juice, unsweetened	50
Tomato juice, canned, no added sugar	46

But, of course, carbs are not the whole story for slimmers. Another vitally important factor is the second major nutrient in our diets – fats. More about those in Chapter 5.

Chapter 4

Can You Eat A Rainbow?

Before we leave carbs, let's take a closer look at the largest group of them – fruit and vegetables. After all, the inclusion of fruit and veg is one of the cardinal differences between this diet and other low carb diets such as Atkin's.

Let me start by asking you: Can you eat a rainbow? If you think the answer is No, let me show you why you might want to rethink your answer. And why it's important to try to eat a rainbow.

Twenty years ago doctors began to realise that fruit and vegetables can help prevent cancers. This is because of the foods' chemicals, known as phytochemicals. In particular, fruits and vegetables with the most vibrant colours seemed to be the most beneficial. One of the best examples is beta carotene, which gives carrots their bright orange colour. With time doctors discovered what were the different pigments contained in each of the foods. They also realised that the health benefits went far beyond cancers – they included the prevention of many other diseases, especially coronary heart disease.

So let's take a look at the health-giving properties of some fruit and vegetables. Let's look at a rainbow of colours.

RED/PINK

These contain lycopenes which help prevent some cancers, especially of the prostate, and phenols.

- ❑ Beetroot
- ❑ Red cabbage
- ❑ Pink grapefruit
- ❑ Guavas
- ❑ Red peppers
- ❑ Radishes
- ❑ Tomatoes
- ❑ Water melon

ORANGE

Contain beta-carotene, perhaps the most well known anti-oxidant which protects body cells from a wide range of diseases and is good for eye and skin health.

- ❑ Apricots
- ❑ Carrots
- ❑ Mangoes
- ❑ Canteloupe melon
- ❑ Sweet potatoes
- ❑ Pumpkin, acorn and butternut squash

ORANGE/YELLOW

Contain beta-cryptoxanthin, another anti-oxidant that prevents cell damage.

- ❑ Yellow grapefruit
- ❑ Lemons
- ❑ Nectarines
- ❑ Oranges
- ❑ Papaya
- ❑ Peaches
- ❑ Pineapple
- ❑ Tangerines

YELLOW/GREEN

Contain lutein and xeazanthin which are good for the eyes by helping to prevent cataracts and macular degeneration – both common causes of blindness.

- ❑ Avocado
- ❑ Courgettes
- ❑ Cucumber
- ❑ Green beans
- ❑ Green and yellow peppers
- ❑ Honeydew melon
- ❑ Cos and Romaine lettuce
- ❑ Kiwi fruit
- ❑ Mustard and cress
- ❑ Spinach

GREEN

Contain sulphoraphane, isothiocyanides and indoles which help the liver get rid of toxins.

- ❑ Beans
- ❑ Broccoli
- ❑ Brussels sprouts
- ❑ Cabbage
- ❑ Cauliflower
- ❑ Globe artichokes
- ❑ Kale
- ❑ Peas
- ❑ Spinach
- ❑ Turnip
- ❑ Courgettes

GREEN/WHITE

Contain alliums which help protect against cancer.

- ❑ Asparagus
- ❑ Celery
- ❑ Endive
- ❑ Leeks
- ❑ Onions
- ❑ Canellini beans
- ❑ Chives
- ❑ Garlic
- ❑ Mushrooms
- ❑ Shallots

BLUE/PURPLE/DARK RED

Contains anthocyanins which prevent blood clots, which helps reduce the risk of coronary heart disease.

- ❑ Red apple skins
- ❑ Beetroot
- ❑ Cherries
- ❑ Red peppers
- ❑ Prunes
- ❑ Aubergine
- ❑ Strawberries
- ❑ Red grapes, red grape juice, red wine
- ❑ Plums
- ❑ Raspberries
- ❑ Blackberries, blackcurrants, blueberries, bilberries

AND THEN

Saving the best to the last, there are soybeans. These contain an abundance of goodies including coumarins, flavonoids, inositol, isoflavones, lignans, phenols, plant sterols, protease inhibitors, saponins, and Omega 3 and Omega 6 oils.

So, go on, eat a rainbow each day!

Chapter 5

Smart Fats, Unsmart Fats

All fats are bad. Right? Of course, that's wrong. As with carbs it's a question of quantity and quality – how much and what kind.

We need some dietary fat for our health. Fats supply essential fatty acids and are important for making available to our bodies the fat-soluble vitamins A, D, E and K.

There are two main kinds of fats and oils, and all fatty foods contain them in different proportions. They are:

1. *Saturated fats.* These are solid at room temperature, and they clog up arteries. Examples of foods containing large quantities of them are fatty meats, poultry skin, and full fat dairy products such as whole milk and cream. Palm and coconut oils are also high in saturates.
2. *Unsaturated fats.* These are oils, which means they are liquid at room temperature. Some oils contain mostly *polyunsaturates*, which are liquid even at refrigerator temperatures. Examples are corn oil, safflower oil, soybean oil, and sunflower oil. One particularly beneficial type of polyunsaturates are *omega-3 fatty acids*, found in oily fish (such as fresh or smoked salmon, mackerel, sardines, herring and white albacore tuna), flaxseed and omega-3 fortified eggs. We'll look at omega-3s in more detail in the next chapter. Other unsaturated oils are *monounsaturates.* These are thick but not completely hard at refrigerator temperatures. They are the healthiest, and are found in nuts (especially almonds, cashews, pistachios, peanuts and peanut butter), olives and olive oil, canola (rapeseed) oil and avocados.

The main concern is the effect of the different kinds of fats and oils on our blood fats and on our hearts. So, a short diversion next about blood fats.

There are two important ones – cholesterol and triglycerides. As regards cholesterol, there are two main types – LDL (which stands for low density lipoprotein), which is the naughty stuff that clogs up our arteries, and HDL (high density lipoprotein), which is the good type that protects our arteries.

Levels of both are affected by diet. HDL is also affected by exercise (which increases it) and smoking (which lowers it).

Triglycerides are also important for lots of health reasons, but especially for our hearts. Too many of them and our risk of coronary heart disease rises.

Saturated fats increase LDL (bad cholesterol) and are bad for the heart. Polyunsaturates lower LDL and, although they unfortunately also lower HDL (good cholesterol), they are good for the heart. Monounsaturates are the best. They both lower LDL and raise HDL, and are very healthy for the heart.

A word about most margarines: these are vegetable oils artificially saturated (hydrogenated) to make them semi-solid. As a result they contain fats called *trans fatty acids* which are probably more harmful even than saturated fats because they increase LDL and lower HDL.

So you can see that the best fats to include in your diet, whether or not you are trying to lose weight, are those with lots of monounsaturates and polyunsaturates (especially omega-3 oils). What are the best ways to achieve this?

- ❑ Avoid fatty meats and poultry skin.
- ❑ Eat oily fish. If you don't like fish consider taking omega-3 fish oil supplements.
- ❑ Drink skimmed, or at the very least semi-skimmed, milk and eat low fat cheeses such as cottage cheese, feta and ricotta.
- ❑ Choose light margarine or margarine that is labelled polyunsaturated and trans-free. Use light margarine instead of butter or ordinary margarine.
- ❑ Use low fat or fat-free mayonnaise and salad dressings.
- ❑ Buy foods that are labelled low fat.
- ❑ Cook with liquid oils rather than solid fats. Especially good are olive and canola (rapeseed) oils. Alternatives are corn oil, peanut and sesame oils.
- ❑ Bake or steam rather than sauté or fry.
- ❑ Eat less commercially prepared baked goods, snack foods, and processed foods, including fast foods.
- ❑ Try to avoid foods containing hydrogenated or partially hydrogenated oils. Or at least choose food products that list the hydrogenated oils near the end of the ingredient list (which means the amount present is likely to be very small).

The advantage of *The Doctor's Diet* compared with popular low carb high protein diets, such as Atkins, is that it encourages good fats (monounsaturates and polyunsaturates) whilst discouraging bad fats (saturated fats and trans fats). The good fats help sugar and insulin metabolism, which helps long-term weight loss, while the bad fats damage sugar and insulin metabolism, which makes weight gain very likely after initial weight loss.

Our diets need a balance of proteins, fats and carbohydrates. In the previous chapter we saw how to choose the good carbs. In this chapter we have seen how to choose the good fats. So don't dismiss carbs and fats. Instead choose smart carbs and smart fats.

Chapter 6

Omega-3 Oils

Time for a science lesson! Essential fatty acids, or EFAs, are so called because our bodies cannot produce them. We need them in our diet. They are important for several reasons, one being that they are used in the manufacture of substances called prostaglandins which are essential for hundreds of bodily functions.

There are two types of EFA:

1. Omega-6 oils, such as linoleic acid, which we get from seed oils such as maize oil and sunflower.
2. Omega-3 oils, which we get from green leafy vegetables eg broccoli, spinach, lettuce; and fish oils such as those we get from mackerel, herring and salmon.

Incidentally, omega-3 oils are particularly important in early life, so that pregnant mums should make sure they have a good intake of these.

A diet rich in animal (or saturated) fats, or too much alcohol, or conditions such as diabetes and virus infections, or getting older, may interfere with the conversion of these oils to prostaglandins. This is why EFA supplements are proving so popular.

EFAs are extremely important for our general health and, for example, for the prevention of heart disease. A good intake of EFAs will ensure a good level of prostaglandins which will maximise the efficiency of the body's various metabolic processes.

Omega-3s are the most interesting and most important, so let's take a closer look at them. There are three types:

- ❑ Alpha-Linolenic acid – which comes from green leafy vegetables, oils, nuts and soybeans;
- ❑ Docosahexanoic acid (DHA) – which comes from oily fish, especially mackerel, sardines, salmon and albacore tuna;
- ❑ Eicosapentanoic acid (EPA) – which also comes from oily fish.

DHA and EPA, the omega-3s from fish, are the most powerful. They are especially important in the prevention and treatment of coronary heart disease, hypertension (high blood pressure), cancer and rheumatoid arthritis.

How do omega-3s help in heart disease? There are several ways they do this:

- They increase levels of HDL (high density lipoprotein) cholesterol. This is the good cholesterol which protects us from coronary heart disease. Remember, there are essentially two different kinds of cholesterol – HDL and LDL. LDL (low density lipoprotein) cholesterol is the bad guy that clogs up our arteries. So we want as little LDL as possible and as much HDL as we can. Three factors which affect cholesterol levels are (1) smoking, (2) lack of exercise, and (3) a poor diet. All three push up LDL and lower HDL – bad news. So anything that lowers LDL and raises HDL is good. Cutting back on animal fats such as fatty meats and dairy products helps as does having a lot of omega-3s.
- Omega-3s, especially the fish ones, push up HDL.
- They lower blood levels of triglycerides – another fat that is a risk factor for coronary heart disease.
- They reduce our risk of developing abnormal heart rhythms which can cause sudden death.
- They help reduce high blood pressure, but only if taken in high quantities through supplements.
- They reduce blood clotting which reduces the risk of clotting inside coronary arteries. This clotting is one important factor in causing heart attacks.

SOME MYTHS ABOUT FATS

There is a lot of confusion about fatty foods – what's good and what's bad.

Let's look at a few of them.

VEGETABLE OILS

A popular myth is that all vegetable oils are good for you. But coconut oil and palm oil are both high in saturated fats, which are the fats that cause high cholesterol. So avoid these and opt instead for oils that are low in saturated fats. Good choices are nut oils, especially peanut, which contain mainly monounsaturated fats which are best for the heart.

Experiment with different oils. For example:

- ❑ As an all-purpose cooking and baking oil use canola (rapeseed) oil. Low in saturated fats, rich in healthy monounsaturated and omega-3 fats, it has a very bland taste. As an alternative use soybean oil which is also bland but contains less omega-3 fat.
- ❑ Try a nutty oil, such as walnut oil, for a salad dressing or baking. Contains a lot of omega-3 fat. Can go rancid quickly, so keep refrigerated after opening.
- ❑ Use olive oil for Mediterranean food and salads. Full of healthy monounsaturates it adds a delicious flavour to foods, especially if you use extra-virgin varieties.
- ❑ For frying and roasting use oils that have little flavour and high smoking points, such as sunflower oil.
- ❑ For stir fries try oils with a distinctive flavour, such as peanut or sesame oil.
- ❑ Nonstick vegetable oil cooking sprays are a good way of providing an almost negligible amount of fat when you need to prevent food from sticking to a pan.

CHEESE

When I worked as a physician in a well known wellness clinic in London I often found myself advising patients about their cholesterol levels. The common reply was: "But I don't eat anything to cause a high cholesterol." A little digging found that, yes, their diet was very healthy except for one thing – they nearly all ate a lot of cheese. So what can you do if cheese is high on your list of life's priorities? Here are some tips:

- ❑ Try lower fat cheeses such as cottage cheese, ricotta and feta.
- ❑ Eat fuller fat cheeses in smaller amounts.
- ❑ Make your fuller fat soft cheeses go a long way by eating them with low fat crackers or fruit or celery sticks.
- ❑ Grating hard cheeses will make them go further.
- ❑ Go for a small amount of a strong-flavoured cheese, such as a Stilton, rather than eating larger amounts of milder-tasting cheeses.

NUTS

Nuts, peanuts, and peanut butter are mostly fat. So should we avoid them?

As we have seen in this chapter there are bad fats but there are also good fats. In 2002 a very interesting piece of research on nuts was published in the prestigious *Journal of the American Medical Association.* Entitled *Nut and peanut butter consumption and risk of type 2 diabetes in women* it showed that women who ate at least five ounces of peanuts and peanut butter a week reduced their risk of developing type 2 diabetes by 21 per cent compared with those who rarely or never ate them. The research also found that women who often ate tree nuts, such almonds, walnuts, cashews, pecans and pistachios, reduced their risk for type 2 diabetes by 27 per cent compared with women who rarely ate them.

But nuts make you put on weight, don't they? Well, do they? In a major piece of research on over 80,000 American nurses over 16 years, scientists found that women who ate the most nuts tended to weigh a bit less and have a lower body mass index than the others.

Nuts and peanuts (which, incidentally are not true nuts but legumes) are rich in the healthy kinds of fats – monounsaturated and polyunsaturated – and both are good sources of antioxidants, protein, magnesium and fibre. They also have a low GI and have good effects on cholesterol and triglyceride levels. Research shows that the more nuts we eat the less our risk of coronary heart disease. If you want to avoid heart disease and diabetes eat more nuts, peanuts and peanut butter instead of fatty meats and refined grains. But, of course, everything in moderation!

Here is a list of the saturated fat and total fat content of some popular nuts:

Nuts (1 oz)	**Saturated Fat (g)**	**Total Fat (g)**
Almonds, dry roasted	1.4g	14.6g
Brazil nuts	4.6g	19.0g
Cashew nuts	2.6g	13.2g
Chestnuts	trace	0.3g
Coconut, dried	16.0g	18.3g
Hazelnuts	1.4g	18.8g
Macadamia nuts	3.1g	21.0g
Mixed nuts, oil-roasted	2.5g	16.0g
Pecans	1.5g	18.3g
Peanuts, dry roasted	2.0g	14.0g
Peanuts, oil-roasted	2.5g	16.0g
Peanuts, boiled (shelled)	1.0g	6.0g
Peanuts, Spanish, raw	2.0g	14.0g
Peanuts, chocolate coated (10)	6g	13.0
Pine nuts	2.2g	14.3g
Pistachios	1.7g	13.7g
Walnuts	1g	16g

Chapter 7

Vitamin Pills

ARE VITAMINS A WASTE OF TIME?

Doctors are split on this one. A lot of the medical press pooh-poohs supplements. But at medical seminars I am always surprised at the number of eminent specialists who secretly admit to taking vitamin pills. I take a variety of supplements. These include B vitamins, especially vitamin B12 and folic acid. Why? Because there is evidence that high blood levels of homocysteine (in the metabolism of which the B-vitamins folate and B12 play a key role) may be a risk factor for Alzheimer's disease and coronary heart disease. There is a considerable difference in death rates from heart disease and stroke between northern and southern European countries. A key difference is the higher consumption of fruit and vegetables in the South. It used to be thought that this protective effect of fruit and vegetables was due to antioxidants. But fruit and vegetables are also one of the main dietary sources of folate which probably has a beneficial effect on the lining of arteries. Taking folic acid supplements over many years may also substantially reduce the risk of breast and bowel cancer.

Selenium is important for the body's immune system – vital to fight infection – and seems to be a key nutrient in stopping HIV progressing to AIDS. It is needed for sperm motility and may reduce the risk of miscarriage. Selenium deficiency has been linked to depression. Selenium and vitamin E may be helpful in reducing heart disease and stroke as well as cancer risk. In particular, research suggests that high selenium and vitamin E intake lowers the risk of prostate cancer. There is some evidence that vitamin E may also be helpful in Alzheimer's disease.

Evidence first reported 20 years ago from the Greenland Inuit population suggested that fatty fish and fish oils contained substances that reduced the incidence of coronary heart disease. These substances – omega-3 fatty acids – were found in early clinical trials to reduce platelet stickiness and to reduce the levels of triglyceride (a blood fat) by as much as 35%. More recent trials have found that omega-3 fatty acids also appear to reduce the risk of abnormal heart rhythms and sudden cardiac death and modestly reduce atherosclerosis plaque formation and high blood pressure. Omega-3 fish oils may also reduce the risk of stroke. Omega-3 oils are good for baby's brain and nerve development in late pregnancy. For a more in depth look at omega-3s look at the previous chapter.

HOW MUCH SHOULD YOU TAKE?

This is difficult to answer. First, not all doctors are convinced of the benefits of supplements. Second, there has not been enough research to give definitive answers. But as a guide let me tell you what I take each day:

Multivitamins	1 tablet
Folic acid	800 micrograms
Vitamin B12	1,000 micrograms
Vitamin E	400 i.u.
Selenium	200 micrograms
Omega-3 (EPA) fish oils	1000 mg x3

But before taking any supplements remember two important points.

1. These are *supplements*. That means they are to be taken *as well as* a healthy balanced diet with its minimum of five portions of fruit and vegetables a day – *not instead of*.
2. Do please first check with your doctor that it is okay for you to take them.

C hapter 8

The Scales – Are They Right?

Before we go much further, it would be useful to decide if we really are overweight and, if so, by how much.

There is no single ideal weight for each height. Instead there is a range of healthy weights based on a measurement called Body Mass Index (BMI). This is calculated by dividing your weight in kilograms (without clothes) by the square of your height in metres (without shoes). Quite complicated to do if maths isn't your favourite subject, so I've done the calculation for you below. For both men and women healthy BMIs are between 20 and 25, and the tables below are based on this range. Weights above and below this range are unhealthy. For someone whose weight is at the upper end of the range there is no *medical* need to lose further weight. As to looking good in your favourite bikini – that's another matter!

WAIST MEASUREMENT

Being overweight is a risk to your health. The height-weight tables give you a good idea of whether you are underweight, normal weight, overweight or obese. But it is not only how much excess weight – or fat – that you are carrying that matters. It is also important to know where in your body that fat is. In particular, fat around your waist carries the greatest risk.

You can find out if you are carrying excess fat in your abdomen by simply measuring your waist circumference. To do this, first stand up. Then find the point which is half-way between the top of your hip bone and the bottom of your rib cage vertically below your armpit. (Incidentally, this is not necessarily where your umbilicus, or belly-button, is.) Then look at the following table:

	Increased risk	**Substantial risk**
Men	94 cm (37 inches) or more	102 cm (40 inches) or more
Women	80 cm (32 inches) or more	88 cm (35 inches) or more

Height	Weight range (feet and inches, stones and pounds)			
	From		To	
ft in	st lb	lb	st lb	lb
4 8	6 6	90	8 0	112
4 9	6 9	93	8 4	116
4 10	6 12	96	8 8	120
4 11	7 1	99	8 12	124
5 0	7 5	103	9 3	129
5 1	7 8	106	9 7	133
5 2	7 12	110	9 11	137
5 3	8 1	113	10 1	141
5 4	8 4	116	10 5	145
5 5	8 8	120	10 10	150
5 6	8 12	124	11 1	155
5 7	9 2	128	11 6	160
5 8	9 6	132	11 11	165
5 9	9 10	136	12 2	170
5 10	10 0	140	12 7	175
5 11	10 4	144	12 12	180
6 0	10 8	148	13 3	185
6 1	10 12	152	13 8	190
6 2	11 2	156	14 0	196
6 3	11 6	160	14 5	201

Height	Weight range (metres and kilograms)	
	From	To
metres	kg	kg
1.40	39	49
1.42	40	50
1.44	42	52
1.46	43	53
1.48	44	55
1.50	45	56
1.52	46	58
1.54	48	60
1.56	49	61
1.58	50	63
1.60	51	64
1.62	52	66
1.64	54	67
1.66	55	69
1.68	56	71
1.70	58	73
1.72	59	74

If your waist circumference is greater than the levels above it is even more important from a health point of view to lose weight. The good news is that the diet in this book is particularly good at helping to get rid of a large tummy – as well as shedding the bits you don't want on your hips and thighs!

HOW OFTEN SHOULD YOU WEIGH YOURSELF?

Most doctors and dieticians will tell you: once a week. Let me tell you why I think that's completely wrong.

I don't believe there is one answer that suits everyone and every situation. For a start, it depends on how much weight you need to lose. And it also depends on whether you're still shedding weight or you're maintaining weight loss. I'll explain.

If you are *very* overweight you will lose weight more quickly than someone with only a few pounds to lose. Also you probably need a lot of motivation and feedback. Why wait a whole week when the likelihood is that you're going to see measurable results every 2-3 days. Now when you get closer to your target weight you'll find that your weight comes off more slowly. At that point weighting yourself once a week makes good sense.

Now let's look at the situation when you've lost your weight and you just want to make sure you don't pile it back on again. Is it easier to lose 1lb or 2lb that you've accidentally gained? Is it easier to lose 2lb or 4lb? Well, the only way to spot that 1lb before it's crept up to 2lb or that 2lb before it's reached 4lb is to weigh yourself every day. Small corrections are much easier to make than large ones.

A final tip: always weigh yourself at the same time of day – ideally as soon as you get out of bed and before you've had breakfast.

Chapter 9

Eating Out

There always comes the day every dieter dreads. I don't mean Christmas or holidays which, yes, may present a challenge. What I have in mind is the day you are invited to go out for a meal in a restaurant. At home you can control what you cook and eat. But in a restaurant? What do you do? Do you ask the waiter, "Is this a GI friendly place?". "Excuse me," comes the reply, "but what is GI?". Your heart sinks. You look at the door and think, should I go now before we've even started? Or do you say to yourself, "Blow the diet, I'll gorge myself for once"?

The good news is, you don't have to do either. It is quite feasible to follow a low GI diet wherever you are. Just remember a few basic principles:

- You can eat any kind of meat so long as it is lean.
- You can eat any grilled fish, seafood or poultry.
- Best cooking methods are grilled, steamed, broiled, roasted or stir-fried.
- Ask for sauces to be served one side so that you control how much you eat.
- If your choice is an omelette or scrambled eggs ask for more egg white and less yolk.
- You can eat most fruit and vegetables but avoid potatoes other than small new ones. The odd one or two potatoes once in a while when you eat out will do you no harm. But try to avoid chips, baked and mashed potatoes.
- Eat salads liberally. Use a light dressing or a little olive oil. Balsamic vinegar is one of my favourites.
- Don't stuff yourself on bread. In fact, avoid it altogether unless it is wholegrain. Again, as with potatoes, the odd slice even of white bread once in a while will do you no harm. Go very easy on the butter – better to avoid it altogether if you can.
- Don't feel that you necessarily have to have a conventional starter, main and dessert. In most restaurants you can ask for two starters followed by, say, a salad. The portions are likely to be smaller and so less calorific.

- If you really can't resist a rich dessert how about sharing one between two?
- Don't be shy about leaving food on your plate. To the inevitable "Didn't you like it?" from the waiter you can smile sweetly and explain that you are on a diet and ask the waiter to pass your compliments to the chef.
- Try not to arrive at the restaurant starving hungry. If you do you are bound to overeat. Have a light healthy low GI snack before you go, such as a portion of fruit. My favourite is a couple of tablespoons of rolled oats.

Now what to do in various types of ethnic restaurants . . .

CHINESE

It comes as a surprise to many that Chinese food presents few challenges because it has plenty of vegetables and is low in fat. If you stick to lean meat, seafood and vegetables, all of which are available in a wide range, and prefer stir-fried to deep-fried food, you won't go far wrong.

Choose:

- clear soups eg wan tun, hot and sour;
- stir-fries with lean meat, poultry, seafood, vegetables and tofu are good;
- steamed fish;
- vegetables;
- noodles with chicken, seafood or vegetable lo mein (in which the noodles are stir-fried along with the other ingredients);
- chop suey (but avoid fried noodles);
- chow mein (again, no fried noodles);
- sauces: black bean, mustard, oyster, Szechuan.

Avoid:

- white rice other than one or two tablespoons. Ask for long grain rice although your chances of getting this in a Chinese restaurant are slim, in which case opt for oriental noodles (egg, rice, or mung bean).

Ask for:

- sauces to be served one side so that you control how much you eat.

ITALIAN

Choose:

- pasta, but ask for it to be *al dente* and eat a small portion as a starter or a side order. Avoid cheese or cream sauces: instead go for tomato-based or seafood-based sauces;

- vegetable soup (minestrone) or bean-based soup (pasta fagioli);
- lean beef;
- veal (but no breadcrumbs);
- grilled chicken;
- seafood.

Pizzas are fine so long as they are thin crust with a minimum of cheese toppings (go for vegetable toppings instead). Avoid bread unless it is semolina bread. Cappuccino is okay but ask for it to be made with skimmed or semi-skimmed milk.

FRENCH

This can be quite a challenge for the low GI diet because of all the butter, cream and cheese, not to mention French bread which has just about the highest GI of all breads. But a lot of French restaurants now offer more Mediterranean style, low GI choices such as:

- consommé;
- chicken and fish Provençal (with tomato sauce);
- chicken and meat stews (with tomato or wine sauces);
- bouillabaisse (seafood stew);
- ratatouille (vegetable stew);
- steamed or poached chicken, seafood and vegetables.

INDIAN

As with Chinese cuisine it surprises many that Indian cuisine is user-friendly to the low GI dieter. Legumes, chicken, fish, vegetables and yoghurt are all good low GI foods. Basmati rice is also good for the diet. The downside with Indian food is that often a lot of fat is used for frying and many sauces have a heavy butter base, so you need to ask for as little fat and butter to be used as possible.

Good choices are:

- lentil or bean soups;
- biryanas (made with basmati rice);
- curries made with chicken, seafood or vegetables (but avoid those made with coconut);
- chicken or lamb kebabs;
- Tandoori chicken or fish (where the main ingredient is marinated in yoghurt and then baked);
- chicken or shrimp Vindaloo.

JAPANESE

The Japanese have long life expectancies, and one factor in this is their food which is very healthy. On a low GI diet you can eat practically anything you like in a Japanese restaurant except for sticky white rice and tinned lychees.

THAI

As with Japanese cuisine you can eat practically anything you like in a Thai restaurant. The spicy recipes usually contain small amounts of meat, seafood or tofu with vegetables.

MEXICAN

Mexican cuisine can be challenging for the low GI dieter. The food is mainly high in starch and fat and low in fruit and vegetables, leading to an overload of both calories and carbs. Go for grilled chicken and seafood, salads and beans. Also fine are fajitas, burritos, tacos and quesadillas made with wholewheat tortillas. Limit the cheese and sour cream or ask if low fat varieties are available.

TAKE-AWAYS

What can you do about these? The short answer is, avoid them. Their fat content is generally high and the bread and rolls used, as in Hamburgers, have very high GIs.

Chapter 10

The Dreaded E-Word

Yes, time now for that dreaded word. Exercise. But listen, if the very idea makes you retch then by all means skip this chapter. It is not *absolutely essential* to exercise to lose weight. But there's no escaping it certainly helps. Whatever diet you are on – cabbage soup, Atkin's, Stone Age, high fibre, low diddlysquat – exercise will always get you there faster.

Let's start with some basics. What goes up must come down. Most people would agree with what is considered a universal truth. Night follows day – another universal truth.

Here is another universal truth: your weight is a balance between the calories you eat and the calories your body burns up. If you eat more calories than you burn, your weight goes up. If you eat fewer calories than you burn, your weight goes down. It's as simple – and as inevitable – as that.

So, to lose weight you need to eat less. As we've seen, this means less fats and less of the wrong kind of carbs. But if you want to supercharge your weight loss you also need to do more physically.

But which is the most effective physical activity for weight loss? It often surprises people when I say walking or gentle cycling. But that doesn't burn many calories, they say. Surely you need to run fast or do a very energetic workout in a gym? No.

Different types of physical activity have different benefits. If you want to become very fit then hard physical activity is best. But it is not so effective for weight loss because the energy comes from carbohydrate stored in the muscles. Since weight loss is about losing fat, physical activity for slimming needs to use energy from stored fat – and this happens only with gentle physical activity.

Our muscles have three different types of fibres. Some use carbohydrates for energy, some use fat, and some use a combination of the two. In high intensity physical activity carbohydrate, stored in the muscles as glycogen, is the most readily available source of energy. It is burned up quickly only to be replaced just as quickly by the next meal. The body's fat stores are almost untouched. But in low intensity physical activity the body uses more fat burning muscles. Fat is sent from the body's fat depots to the muscles to be burned for fuel.

Good forms of low intensity fat-burning physical activity are walking, cycling and swimming. Others include golf and bowling.

HOW MANY CALORIES CAN I BURN UP DURING PHYSICAL ACTIVITY?

This depends on the physical activity. Here are some examples of calories burned during 30 minutes of physical activity:

	calories
Slow walking (2 mph)	90
Medium pace walking (3 mph)	135
Brisk walking (4 mph)	180
Jogging	300
Cycling (10 mph)	240
Swimming (33 yd/min)	210
Tennis (singles)	210
Typical physical activity video	220
Light gardening	120
Heavy gardening (digging)	240
Skipping (rope)	300

But, remember, low-intensity physical activity, such as slow walking, mobilises more fat (as opposed to carbohydrate) compared with high-intensity physical activity. Low-intensity physical activity is when the heart rate is around 70% of maximum capacity. To work this out, subtract your age from 220 and multiply by 0.7.

For example, if you are 30:
Subtract 30 from 220 = 190
Multiply 190 by 0.7 = 133

Your heart rate during low-intensity physical activity is 133 beats a minute (or 22 beats each 10 seconds). Target low-intensity physical activity heart rates are:

Age	Heart rate/minute	Heart rate/10 seconds
20	140	23
25	137	23
30	133	22
35	130	22
40	126	21
45	123	20
50	119	20
55	116	19
60	112	19
65	109	18
70	105	17

Now, if you stuck out this chapter so far, do remember there are lots of other ways of burning off calories, or body fat (same thing, really) other than formal exercise or workouts. For example, use stairs instead of lifts and escalators. If you use the bus to get home why not leave the bus one stop early and walk the rest of the way? How far away is your corner shop? Could you walk rather than jump in your car? And what better way for a family to spend a couple of hours on a Sunday than to ride bicycles in quiet country lanes or in a park?

In a moment we'll talk a little more about how vigorous exercise should be. But first, it's worth spending a few moments considering the health benefits of exercise apart from weight control. Most people are aware that exercise is 'good' for you in a general sense. But is there actually any scientific evidence for this? Two recent studies shed light on the matter.

The first is the Honolulu Heart Program which followed up 707 non-smoking retired men of Japanese ancestry aged 45 to 68. On average they walked 1.8 miles each day. The death rate over 12 years was analysed according to whether the men walked less than 1 mile, 1 to 2 miles, or more than 2 miles each day. There was no difference between the three groups in terms of weight, diet, alcohol consumption, blood pressure, diabetes or cholesterol. Those who walked less than 1 mile daily were 1.8 times more likely to die of heart disease, stroke, cancer and other causes of death. An interesting way of looking at it is: for every 5 men who walked more than 2 miles a day, one fewer will die over 12 years compared with those who walked less than 1 mile a day.

But is what happens to Japanese men relevant to what happens to men and women in Europe? To answer that let's look at another recent study. The Finnish twin cohort study examined the activity levels and death rates of just under 8,000 male twins and 8,000 female twins. It classified Activity levels as either sedentary (no leisure physical activity), occasional exercise (physical activity less than six times a month) or conditioning exercise (vigorous walking or jogging or comparable activity at least six times a month for an average of 30 minutes). Over 17 years the death rate was 12% for those who were sedentary, 7.4% for occasional exercisers, and 4.9% for conditioning exercisers.

So, the Hawaiian study shows that walking two miles a day reduces the risk of death by nearly a half; the Finnish study shows a reduced risk for moderate exercisers of nearly 60% – a similar result. Could this provide you with additional motivation to exercise which will, of course, have the added benefit of helping your weight control?

Before we leave the E-word let's take another look at the question, 'How vigorous does exercise have to be for weight loss?'. The traditional wisdom was that exercise had to be vigorous and last for at least 20 minutes at least three times a week. Anything less and you might just as well throw away your Nikes and become a couch potato. But recently doubt has been cast on this. A good example is some research described in the January 1999 issue of the International Journal of Obesity. The study compared the effects of diet without exercise, diet with traditional exercise (vigorous activities for 20 minutes three times a week), and diet with the new recommendation for exercise (moderate exercise for 30 minutes five times a week).

Over 16 weeks, the diet alone group lost 6.5 kg (14 lb), the vigorous exercise group lost 11.9 kg (26 lb), and the moderate exercise group lost 10.1 kg (22 lb). The monthly weight loss was just under 4 lb (diet alone), just over 8 lb (vigorous exercise), and 6.6 lb (moderate exercise).

The results underline the value of exercise in weight control. But they also demonstrate that there is little difference in weight loss between those taking vigorous exercise three times a week and those doing moderate physical activity five times a week. Which is good news for most of us. So, have a go. There are lots of fun ways of getting physically more active. And it really does pay.

Chapter 11

Time for More Motivation

Everyone reading this book will have a different target weight. Some will want to lose a lot – some a little. Interestingly, the very people who most need to lose weight are often the ones who fail because they never even start. They look at how much they need to lose to reach a 'normal' weight, and the task is so daunting they give up straightaway. And yet, the benefits of losing even a moderate amount of excess body weight are tremendous. Maintaining a moderate weight loss brings about significant health benefits.

What are these benefits? A weight loss of 5 to 10 kg (11 to 22 lb), or 5 to 10% of body weight, reduces the risk of developing high blood pressure. In people with high blood pressure each kilogram of weight loss produces a fall in blood pressure of between 1 and 2 points. A weight loss of 10% lessens the risk or delays the onset not only of high blood pressure but of high blood cholesterol and type 2 (non-insulin dependent) diabetes. A moderate weight loss also reduces the risk of developing coronary heart disease and stroke. Research has shown that a weight loss of 10 kg reverses the fatty narrowing of coronary arteries without the use of cholesterol-lowering prescription drugs.

Premature death from disease is reduced by at least 20%, with at least a 30% reduction in diabetes-related deaths and more than 40% reduction in deaths from obesity-related cancers (breast, uterus, ovary, cervix and gallbladder). Type 2 diabetes, which is often obesity-related, is a particular concern to doctors because it increases the risk of coronary heart disease and damage to the eyes, kidneys and nerves. Life expectancy of middle-aged people with this type of diabetes is reduced by 5 to 10 years. The good news is that life expectancy is increased by 3 to 4 months for each kilogram of weight lost.

A weight loss of 5 to 10% improves back and joint pain and breathlessness and reduces the frequency of sleep apnoea (the condition in which heavy snorers stop breathing for prolonged periods).

Interestingly, in the USA, nearly 8% of national health-care budgets are linked to obesity and all its complications. This compares with around 5% for type 2 diabetes and 7% for cancer.

So, the message is clear. It doesn't matter how severely overweight you are. Unless you are already within 10 kg of a BMI of 25, aim to lose at least 5 to 10 kg and to maintain this weight loss. If you lose no more you will reap enormous health benefits.

Chapter 12

Store Cupboard and Cooking

WHAT SHOULD YOU KEEP IN YOUR STORE CUPBOARD?

DAIRY PRODUCTS

These are good for the low GI diet because the sugar they contain, which is lactose, is absorbed quite slowly into the blood stream. Especially good for weight control are the low fat versions. So find a place for:

- Milk: skimmed or semi-skimmed; alternatively try soya milk;
- Yoghurt: plain or flavoured low fat or non fat;
- Cheese: low or non fat versions (less than 5g fat per ounce (28g)) of cottage cheese, ricotta cheese, feta cheese, cream cheese, mozzarella cheese, Swiss cheeses, Cheddar cheese; Parmesan cheese for sprinkling on other foods;
- Low fat ice creams and sorbets;
- Spreads: light butter or light margarine; avoid hydrogenated kinds;
- Oils, mayonnaise and salad dressing;
- Oils: canola (rapeseed), olive oil, soybean oil, walnut oil, non-stick vegetable oil cooking spray;
- Mayonnaise: light or non fat;
- Salad dressings: low fat or non fat.

EGGS

- Eggs are not the villains they used to be considered. They contain no saturated fat and raise the good cholesterol more than the bad. And eggs also contain nutrients that may help lower the risk for heart disease, including protein, vitamins B12, D and E, riboflavin, and folate. So eggs are permissible. Up to seven egg yolks a week is fine. But if you have diabetes you should probably limit yourself to no more than two or three eggs a week, as the Nurses' Health Study found that for diabetics an egg a day might increase the risk for heart disease. Also, if you have difficulty controlling your blood cholesterol you need to be careful about eating egg yolks and you should choose foods made with egg whites instead. For everyone, egg whites are unlimited. If you can find them, choose omega-3 enriched eggs.

MEAT, POULTRY AND FISH

- ❑ Lean cuts of all meats. Trim off visible fat.
- ❑ Back bacon.
- ❑ Any fresh or frozen fish or shellfish, but try especially to include oily fish such as salmon.
- ❑ Any tinned fish in water or brine, eg tuna. Avoid fish tinned in oil.

BREADS

Avoid breads, bagels, burger buns and muffins made from finely ground flour. Best to eat are:

- ❑ 100 per cent stone-ground whole wheat bread;
- ❑ Pumpernickel;
- ❑ Multigrain breads;
- ❑ Rye bread;
- ❑ Pita bread;
- ❑ Wholewheat flour tortillas;
- ❑ Sourdough bread, which has a moderately low GI because of its acidity.

PASTA AND NOODLES

- ❑ All pastas are fine providing you cook them *al dente* and you eat small portions, eg 50g, only.
- ❑ Noodles too are fine.

RICE AND OTHER GRAINS

Avoid sticky white rice. Instead choose:

- ❑ Long grain rice, brown rice, long grain brown rice, basmati rice, parboiled or Uncle Ben's converted rice (rice that has been steamed prior to milling);
- ❑ Buckwheat – used, for example, in *kasha*;
- ❑ Barley – used in casseroles, pilaffs and soups;

- Bulgur wheat (cracked wheat) – used in many dishes including casseroles and pilaffs;
- Couscous;
- Polenta (cornmeal).

LEGUMES

- Black beans, kidney beans, chickpeas (eg in hummus), soy beans.

FLOURS

- Whole grain flours;
- Flour alternatives eg wheat germ, wheat bran, oat bran, rolled oats, flaxseeds.

BREAKFAST CEREALS

All Bran, bran buds, muesli, nutri-grain, shredded wheat, Special K, porridge made with rolled grains (not instant porridge).

TINNED FOODS

- Tuna in brine;
- Salmon or sardines in water;
- Sweetcorn;
- Fruits.

CONDIMENTS AND HERBS

- Condiments and herbs are all OK but use tomato ketchup in moderation.

FRUIT AND VEGETABLES

- Most fruit and vegetables are OK except potatoes (other than small new and sweet potatoes), parsnips, carrots (other than small portions) and watermelon. Eat at least 5 portions a day.
- Dried apricots are fine.

NUTS AND SEEDS

- Almonds, pecans, pine nuts, walnuts;
- Peanuts and peanut butter (in small amounts – remember it is quite calorific);
- Flax seeds, sesame seeds, sunflower seeds.

COOKING TIPS

- ❑ Pastas: cook *al dente*. Include vegetables in pasta recipes.
- ❑ Breaded coatings: use Special K rather than breadcrumbs.
- ❑ Meat: use lean cuts. Trim off visible fat. Cooking methods: grill, stir fry, oven fry, bake.
- ❑ Poultry: remove skin. Cooking methods: grill, stir fry, oven fry, bake.
- ❑ Omelettes: use more egg whites, lean meats, lower fat cheeses and lots of vegetables.
- ❑ Casseroles: use basmati, long-grain, converted or wild rice or bulgur wheat instead of white rice. Use lower fat cheeses or sour cream. Include plenty of legumes and vegetables. Use as little oil, butter or margarine as possible.
- ❑ Soups: use basmati, long-grain, converted or wild rice or barley instead of white rice. Include plenty of legumes, vegetables and pasta. Use skimmed or semi-skimmed rather than whole milk. Thicken with puréed vegetables rather than cream.
- ❑ Burgers, meatballs: use extra lean meat. Use cooked lentils, legumes, rolled oats, oat bran or bulgur wheat instead of white rice or bread crumbs. Include lots of chopped vegetables.
- ❑ Stuffings: use low GI breads and lots of chopped vegetables.
- ❑ Sauces: use skimmed or semi-skimmed rather than whole milk. Use as little butter or margarine as possible.
- ❑ Marinades: use more fruit juices with less sugar for sweetness.
- ❑ Salads: use low fat mayonnaise and dressings or sour cream. Use lean meats and lower fat cheeses.
- ❑ Pancakes and Yorkshire pudding batter: use oats, oat bran, wheat bran, wheat germ or flax meal instead of some of the flour. Serve pancakes with low sugar fruit sauce or apple sauce or fruit (fresh or tinned).
- ❑ Custards and puddings: use skimmed or semi skimmed rather than whole milk. Use vanilla, cinnamon or nutmeg instead of some or all of the sugar.
- ❑ Sandwiches: use low GI breads and lots of vegetables.

FINALLY, THE 'MAGIC FOOD'

There is one food which is becoming very popular today but which has been around for centuries. What is it? Soy.

Is soy just a fad, or is there something more to it?

Soy is what we call soybeans or foods containing part of the soybean. Soy foods belong to the legume/dry bean family. Soy is cholesterol free and low in saturated fat. It is high in protein and fibre and is a good source of calcium, iron, magnesium, and several B vitamins. It also contains linolenic acid, a polyunsaturated omega-3 fatty acid which helps prevent coronary heart disease. The American FDA has stated that diets containing 25 grams of soy protein and low saturated fat each day can decrease cholesterol. This in turn helps prevent coronary heart disease. This beneficial effect of soy is due to the presence of genistein, a natural oestrogenic compound which significantly lowers levels of LDL cholesterol (the bad cholesterol) and triglycerides while increasing levels of HDL cholesterol (the good cholesterol). Genistein occurs naturally in soy and in no other food.

Soy contains antioxidants (compounds that prevent body cell damage caused by unstable oxygen molecules called 'free radicals'). Cell damage leads on to cancer formation as well as premature aging. Women who eat soy are much less likely to develop breast cancer than those who don't. Similarly there is a much lower incidence of prostate cancer amongst men who eat soy products such as tofu. The genistein found in soy reduces the severity of menopausal hot flushes.

Soy is high in fibre and for this reason may help prevent cancer of the stomach and bowel. Soy's protein and fibre help regulate blood glucose levels. This means that soy is likely to be of benefit in obesity and diabetes. It lowers blood lipids, such as cholesterol, and reduces insulin and insulin resistance. Soy's protein enhances the body's ability to retain and absorb calcium in the bones. This improves bone density which may help prevent thinning of bones and osteoporosis.

Most important of all for this book's diet, soybeans have the lowest GI values of any food. Add them to your other food and you will reduce the glycaemic index of your meal.

WHAT ARE THE WAYS TO INCORPORATE SOY IN YOUR DIET?

Apart from whole soybeans, foods containing soybeans include soy milk, soy yoghurt, soy nut butter, soy flour, tofu, soy nuts and meat analogs (for example, burgers and nuggets that look and taste like meat, poultry, or fish).

Here are some ways to incorporate soy in your diet:

- ❑ In cooking, replace cow's milk with soy milk.
- ❑ Blend soy milk with fruit juice or fruit for a healthy nutritious drink.

- Use soy milk instead of cow's milk on your breakfast cereal or use it instead of cow's milk or water to make porridge. In fact, you can use soy milk whenever you like as a cow's milk substitute – for example, in cream sauces, soups, custards, shakes, and batter and pancake or waffle mixes.
- Use soy flour to thicken gravies and cream sauces.
- Canned soybeans are available as regular or black soybeans and are good substitutes with lots of flavour for other beans in any recipe.
- Use textured soy protein (TSP) or textured vegetable protein (TVP), made from soy flour, as a substitute for meat in stews and casseroles. When mixed with water, TSP has a texture similar to ground beef and can be used partially to replace it in spaghetti sauce, chilli or meatloaf.
- Soy nuts have less fat than ordinary nuts so provide a useful low fat snack and they work well in salads. If you can find soy nut butter this is an excellent alternative to peanut butter.
- If you can find it use okara, the soybean pulp by-product of soy milk, as a thickener.
- Add tofu, a very mild flavoured soy food with the texture of ricotta cheese, to soups, casseroles and stir-fries to act as a flavour sponge.

Tofu is a very interesting soy product. It is made from soymilk to which a coagulating agent is added to separate the liquid into curds and whey – similar to making cheese. The curds are then pressed into a solid block, stored in water and either refrigerated or vacuum-packed. It is available in a variety of textures ranging from extra firm to firm to soft to silken. Extra firm tofu keeps its shape well and is best for slicing, dicing and frying, and broiling. It can be frozen then thawed, which gives it a chewy texture similar to meat, and is ideal stir-fried with vegetables or added to casseroles, chilli, lasagne, or used as a spaghetti sauce. If you cut it into cubes you can use it as a kebab on a barbecue.

Firm tofu, being less dense, is useful for dressings, desserts and as a substitute for soft cheeses such as cream, cottage or ricotta.

Soft tofu is even less dense and is good for puréed dishes and for blending into dressings and sauces or with fruit to make delicious smoothies. It is useful as an alternative to sour cream or yoghurt. If you'd prefer to have fewer eggs you can reduce the number used in a recipe by substituting tofu for some of the eggs.

Silken tofu is the least dense and is a creamy, custard-like product that is superb in salad dressings, mayonnaise, dips, creamy sauces, cheesecakes and cream pies.

I think it is hard to ignore all the scientific evidence for the benefits of soy, which is why I would encourage you to find ways of incorporating it in your diet.

THE DIET IN A NUTSHELL

Now you have sufficient information to understand the principles of the diet. In a nutshell these are:

Eat:

- ❑ lean meats
- ❑ plenty of fish and seafood
- ❑ low fat dairy products
- ❑ low GI wholegrain breads and cereal
- ❑ low GI rice
- ❑ small portions of pasta cooked *al dente*
- ❑ plenty of low GI fruit and vegetables
- ❑ plenty of beans, peas and lentils
- ❑ monounsaturated and omega-3-rich oils eg olive and canola (rapeseed) oils
- ❑ more soya products

Chapter 13

Orientation Phase

Time now to get down to business. You've read all the whys and wherefores of this book's diet. And if you haven't read them you could struggle. Why? Because this diet is going to be a little different to what you're used to. And unless you really understand why you may have to go without *some* of the foods you are used to but in their place you can and should eat foods which you hadn't previously thought about but which are *equally delicious*, you may become demotivated. And that could lead to failure.

So, just in case you decided to skip the book to this point, allow me to do a quick recap. This diet is completely different to other popular diets such as low fat and high protein/low carb diets. Its basis is that to lose weight you need to watch not only fats but carbs. But please note: *watch* carbs, *not* cut them out! It's the quality of the carbs that counts. The *wrong* carbs make your body pump out lots of insulin which pushes fat into your body's cells and stops that fat from getting out again. The *right* carbs encourage your body to burn off fat and satisfy your hunger for much longer so that you end up eating less.

So this diet is about eating the right foods, which means a healthy balance of proteins, fats and the right carbs, and preparing or cooking that food in a way which doesn't encourage your body to lay down fat. If you follow the advice *you will lose weight.* Equally important, you will enjoy good tasty food and you won't be hungry. And the icing on the cake, if you'll forgive an inappropriate metaphor in a book on diet, is that you'll reap health benefits – less likelihood of developing coronary heart disease or diabetes.

So let's start at the beginning. Like all good (and bad) diet books there are two phases to the diet – Orientation (phase 1) and Continuation (phase 2). Why? Simply because most of us who have quite a bit of weight to shed need a kick start. If you lose only a pound in your first week you might become demotivated. But lose 4 or 5 pounds or more and you'll feel that you've hit the ground running. You'll feel that you really are well on the road towards your target.

Of course not all that initial weight loss will be fat – some of it will be fluid. That happens on *every* diet no matter whether it is low fat, high protein, or good old fashioned starvation. But soon all your weight loss will be fat.

The other reason for an Orientation phase is that it's a useful phase to return to in future if you've been a bit 'naughty' and put on weight again – perhaps because of Christmas or a holiday.

Orientation lasts for 2 weeks. As you'd expect, there are tighter guidelines as to what you can and can't eat. Then after 2 weeks you go on to Continuation. This lasts for the rest of your life. But remember, you will enjoy Continuation. (You'll enjoy Orientation but Continuation will be that much more fun.) You're going to be eating lots of wonderful tasty foods and you won't be feeling hungry. Enjoy!

For each phase you will find 2 weeks' of suggested menus for every meal. I strongly suggest that in Orientation, at least, you stick as closely as you can to those suggestions. But if you find there is a food that you really don't like then by all means substitute that meal suggestion with another. It is important that you enjoy the diet from the very start. The menus for Orientation follow in the next chapter.

SO, WELCOME TO ORIENTATION

What can you expect? As you will have come to expect by now, you'll find lots of suggestions for a healthy, nutritious, delicious, well balanced diet. You will find too that there are carbs, but not as many as you will have once you go on to Continuation. The list of foods for Orientation is on the next two pages.

PHASE 1: ORIENTATION. FOODS TO INCLUDE AND FOODS TO AVOID

	FOODS TO INCLUDE	**FOODS TO AVOID**
ALCOHOL		All alcohol
BREADS		All breads
CEREALS		All cereals

	FOODS TO INCLUDE	**FOODS TO AVOID**
CHEESE	Low fat cottage cheese	Medium and high fat cheeses eg:
	Any low fat version of other cheeses	Brie
	Feta	Edam
	Mozzarella	Stilton
	Parmesan	
	Ricotta	
COOKING OIL	Canola oil (rapeseed oil)	
	Olive oil	
DAIRY	Skimmed milk	Whole or semi-skimmed milk
	Soya milk	Yoghurt, non low-fat
	Low-fat yoghurts, plain and fruit	Ice cream
EGGS	Yolks: as you like, but follow any medical advice you may have been given	
	Whites: unlimited	
ETHNIC	Hummus	
	Mexican wheat tortillas	
FRUIT	Apricots, dried Cherries Grapefruit, fresh – 3 TIMES A DAY! Prunes	All except in left hand column
FRUIT JUICES	Tomato juice	All juices except in left hand column
	Lemon juice, lime juice	

	FOODS TO INCLUDE	**FOODS TO AVOID**
LENTILS	Butter beans	
	Chickpeas	
	Kidney beans	
	Lentils	
	Soya beans	
MEAT	Lean cuts with no visible fat of:	All fatty meats and visible fat
	Beef	Liver
	Pork including ham and bacon	
	Veal	
NUTS	All, but daily limits:	
	Brazils 10	
	Cashews 15	
	Peanuts 20	
	Peanut butter – 15g (1 tablespoon)	
	Pistachios 30	
	Walnuts 15	
PASTA		All pasta
POULTRY	White meat without skins:	Poultry red meat:
	Chicken breast	Chicken wings and legs
	Turkey breast	Turkey wings and legs
		Chicken liver
		Duck
		Goose
RICE		All rice

	FOODS TO INCLUDE	**FOODS TO AVOID**
SEAFOOD	All fish and shellfish	
SPICES & SAUCES	All non-sugared sauces and spices (check the labels)	
	Horseradish sauce	
	Pepper	
VEGETABLES	All green vegetables	All except in left hand column
	Artichokes	
	Cauliflower	
	Aubergine	
	Mushrooms	
	Onions	
	Peppers	
	Radishes	
	Tomatoes	
MISCELLANEOUS	Horseradish sauce	Tomato ketchup
	Pepper	
	Salt – as little as possible	
	Soy sauce	
	Worcestershire sauce	

	FOODS TO INCLUDE	FOODS TO AVOID
DRINKS	Tea*	Excess coffee
	Coffee* (2 cups a day)	Non low calorie soft drinks
	Decaffeinated coffee (unlimited)	Excess low calorie soft drinks unless caffeine-free
	Low calorie soft drinks (limit 2 drinks a day unless caffeine-free)	
	* Tea and coffee to be drunk preferably black or with a dash of skimmed or soya milk; no sugar (but artificial sweetener allowed)	

TIME TO START!

But first, a word or two about the 14 day Orientation menus and recipes.

- ❑ The recipes are generally simple and quick. This is in order to help keep you out of the kitchen as much as possible. In particular, the evening meal has the minimum of preparation time and washing up.
- ❑ The number of vegetables is kept to a minimum – generally just one!
- ❑ You are encouraged to drink a lot of water. There are many reasons for this. Two important ones are:

1. Lack of water causes dehydration even if you don't feel thirsty. And dehydration makes you tired and lethargic and less enthusiastic about everything – including your diet!
2. Water fills your stomach up and helps you to feel satisfied with less food.

GRAPEFRUIT

And now for the most important point: grapefruit. You've heard of the Grapefruit Diet. Unless you've been living all your life on a desert island you cannot fail to have read about it. It's been around a long time – since the 1930s in fact. And various incarnations of it seem to have worked to some extent. But the problem has always been that the diet has been too restrictive for people to follow indefinitely. And, until recently, no-one has understood why grapefruit can help weight loss.

Recently a paper was published which reported the results of a 12-week study carried out on 100 obese people in the USA. One group ate half of a grapefruit three times a day before each meal. Another drank a glass of grapefruit juice before every meal. A third did not include grapefruit in their meals. The group eating grapefruit without otherwise changing their diet lost an average of 3.6 pounds, some shedding as much as 10 pounds. The group drinking grapefruit juice, again without otherwise changing their diet, lost an average of 3.3 pounds. The control group, who consumed no grapefruit, lost an average of only 0.5 pounds.

Measurement of glucose levels led the researchers to believe that the weight loss was probably linked to lowered levels of insulin. Insulin is used to metabolise sugar. The more efficiently sugar is metabolised, the less likely it is to be stored as fat in the body. Also, lowering insulin levels makes you feel less hungry. High levels of insulin cause hunger and also stimulate the liver to manufacture fat that increases body weight and also causes coronary heart disease.

The inclusion of grapefruit at each meal helps weight loss, reduces the risk of coronary heart disease, and lowers the risk of developing type 2 diabetes. (But please see the warning about grapefruit interactions at the end of this book.)

All of which fits in so well with *The Doctor's Diet.* In fact, for slimmers, grapefruit and *The Doctor's Diet* are an immensely powerful combination.

So the plan is, in the Orientation phase, you eat half a grapefruit before each of your three main meals each day. Of course, you can carry this on into the Maintenance phase. Indeed if you still have weight to lose after Orientation it is important that you do continue with grapefruit.

In the next chapter you will find menus for each of the 14 days of the Orientation Phase. You will find recipes for items marked with a * in Chapter 15.

Enjoy!
Enjoy reading.
Enjoy losing weight.
Enjoy your food.

Chapter 14

Orientation Phase Daily Menus

Menus for Day 1

Breakfast

- ❑ A glass of water
- ❑ Half a grapefruit (with optional artificial sweetener)
- ❑ An egg poached in water with a splash of vinegar with 2 rashers of grilled lean back bacon
- ❑ Tea or decaffeinated coffee with optional skimmed milk and sweetener but no sugar

Morning Snack

- ❑ A glass of water
- ❑ 5 Brazil nuts*
  (*or 1 oz flax seeds, sesame seeds or sunflower seeds. If you wish, use seeds as alternatives to nuts throughout the menus)

Lunch

- ❑ A glass of water
- ❑ Half a grapefruit (with optional artificial sweetener)
- ❑ 4 heaped soup spoons of cottage cheese, sprinkled with 2 chopped dried apricots

Afternoon Snack

- ❑ A glass of water
- ❑ A bowl of cherries

Dinner

- ❑ A glass of water
- ❑ Half a grapefruit (with optional artificial sweetener)
- ❑ Herb chicken with green vegetables*
- ❑ Ricotta cheese dessert*
  or plain or fruit low fat yoghurt
  or a small bowl of cherries or 4 dried apricots
  or either the yoghurt or fruit with sugar-free jelly
- ❑ Tea or decaffeinated coffee with optional skimmed milk and sweetener but no sugar

Menus for Day 2

Breakfast

- A glass of water
- Half a grapefruit (with optional artificial sweetener)
- Low fat fruit yoghurt
- Tea or decaffeinated coffee with optional skimmed milk and sweetener but no sugar

Morning Snack

- A glass of water
- Celery stick stuffed with any low fat cheese such as cottage cheese, Laughing Cow light cheese

Lunch

- A glass of water
- Half a grapefruit (with optional artificial sweetener)
- Mixed green salad – as much as you want

Afternoon Snack

- A glass of water
- 8 cashew nuts

Dinner

- A glass of water
- Half a grapefruit (with optional artificial sweetener)
- A glass of tomato juice
- Pork medallion fillets with green vegetables*
- Ricotta cheese dessert*
  or plain or fruit low fat yoghurt
  or a small bowl of cherries or 4 dried apricots
  or either the yoghurt or fruit with sugar-free jelly
- Tea or decaffeinated coffee with optional skimmed milk and sweetener but no sugar

Menus for Day 3

Breakfast

- ❑ A glass of water
- ❑ Half a grapefruit
- ❑ 2 egg omelette with 2 rashers of grilled back bacon
- ❑ Tea or decaffeinated coffee with optional skimmed milk and sweetener but no sugar

Morning Snack

- ❑ A glass of water
- ❑ 10 peanuts, unsalted

Lunch

- ❑ A glass of water
- ❑ Half a grapefruit (with optional artificial sweetener)
- ❑ 75 g lean diced ham
- ❑ Mixed green salad – as much as you want

Afternoon Snack

- ❑ A glass of water
- ❑ Celery stick with hummus

Dinner

- ❑ A glass of water
- ❑ Half a grapefruit (with optional artificial sweetener)
- ❑ A glass of tomato juice
- ❑ Cod fish grill with broccoli*
- ❑ Ricotta cheese dessert*
  or plain or fruit low fat yoghurt
  or a small bowl of cherries or 4 dried apricots
  or either the yoghurt or fruit with sugar-free jelly
- ❑ Tea or decaffeinated coffee with optional skimmed milk and sweetener but no sugar

Menus for Day 4

Breakfast

- ❑ A glass of water
- ❑ Half a grapefruit (with optional artificial sweetener)
- ❑ Low fat fruit yoghurt
- ❑ Tea or decaffeinated coffee with optional skimmed milk and sweetener but no sugar

Morning Snack

- ❑ A glass of water
- ❑ Celery stick stuffed with any low fat cheese such as cottage cheese, Laughing Cow light cheese

Lunch

- ❑ A glass of water
- ❑ Half a grapefruit (with optional artificial sweetener)
- ❑ 100 g white tuna fish – in brine or water, only
- ❑ Mixed green salad – as much as you want

Afternoon Snack

- ❑ A glass of water
- ❑ 8 walnuts

Dinner

- ❑ A glass of water
- ❑ Half a grapefruit (with optional artificial sweetener)
- ❑ A glass of tomato juice
- ❑ Oriental beef stir fry*
- ❑ Ricotta cheese dessert*
  or plain or fruit low fat yoghurt
  or a small bowl of cherries or 4 dried apricots
  or either the yoghurt or fruit with sugar-free jelly
- ❑ Tea or decaffeinated coffee with optional skimmed milk and sweetener but no sugar

Menus for Day 5

Breakfast

- A glass of water
- Half a grapefruit (with optional artificial sweetener)
- Low fat plain yoghurt
- Tea or decaffeinated coffee with optional skimmed milk and sweetener but no sugar

Morning Snack

- A glass of water
- A bowl of cherries

Lunch

- A glass of water
- Half a grapefruit (with optional artificial sweetener)
- 100 g grilled chicken breast with skin and fat removed
- Mixed green salad – as much as you want

Afternoon Snack

- A glass of water
- 4 dried apricots

Dinner

- A glass of water
- Half a grapefruit (with optional artificial sweetener)
- A glass of tomato juice
- Veal escalope with French beans*
- Ricotta cheese dessert*
  or plain or fruit low fat yoghurt
  or a small bowl of cherries or 4 dried apricots
  or either the yoghurt or fruit with sugar-free jelly
- Tea or decaffeinated coffee with optional skimmed milk and sweetener but no sugar

Menus for Day 6

Breakfast

- ❑ A glass of water
- ❑ Half a grapefruit (with optional artificial sweetener)
- ❑ 2 scrambled eggs with 2 rashers of grilled lean back bacon
- ❑ Tea or decaffeinated coffee with optional skimmed milk and sweetener but no sugar

Morning Snack

- ❑ A glass of water
- ❑ Celery stick stuffed with any low fat cheese such as cottage cheese, Laughing Cow light cheese

Lunch

- ❑ A glass of water
- ❑ Half a grapefruit (with optional artificial sweetener)
- ❑ Gazpacho*
- ❑ Low fat fruit yoghurt

Afternoon Snack

- ❑ A glass of water
- ❑ 8 cashew nuts

Dinner

- ❑ A glass of water
- ❑ Half a grapefruit (with optional artificial sweetener)
- ❑ A glass of tomato juice
- ❑ Fillet of beef steak with asparagus* accompanied by a small bowl of green salad
- ❑ Ricotta cheese dessert*
  or plain or fruit low fat yoghurt
  or a small bowl of cherries or 4 dried apricots
  or either the yoghurt or fruit with sugar-free jelly
- ❑ Tea or decaffeinated coffee with optional skimmed milk and sweetener but no sugar

Menus for Day 7

Breakfast

- ❑ A glass of water
- ❑ Half a grapefruit (with optional artificial sweetener)
- ❑ Low fat fruit yoghurt
- ❑ Tea or decaffeinated coffee with optional skimmed milk and sweetener but no sugar

Morning Snack

- ❑ A glass of water
- ❑ 15 pistachio nuts

Lunch

- ❑ A glass of water
- ❑ 4 heaped soup spoons of cottage cheese
- ❑ Mixed green salad – as much as you want

Afternoon Snack

- ❑ A glass of water
- ❑ Celery stick with hummus

Dinner

- ❑ A glass of water
- ❑ Half a grapefruit (with optional artificial sweetener)
- ❑ A glass of tomato juice
- ❑ Turkey curry* accompanied by green beans
- ❑ Ricotta cheese dessert*
  or plain or fruit low fat yoghurt
  or a small bowl of cherries or 4 dried apricots
  or either the yoghurt or fruit with sugar-free jelly
- ❑ Tea or decaffeinated coffee with optional skimmed milk and sweetener but no sugar

Menus for Day 8

Breakfast

- ❑ A glass of water
- ❑ Half a grapefruit (with optional artificial sweetener)
- ❑ 2 egg omelette with 2 rashers of grilled lean back bacon
- ❑ Tea or decaffeinated coffee with optional skimmed milk and sweetener but no sugar

Morning Snack

- ❑ A glass of water
- ❑ Celery stick stuffed with any low fat cheese such as cottage cheese, Laughing Cow light cheese

Lunch

- ❑ A glass of water
- ❑ Half a grapefruit (with optional artificial sweetener)
- ❑ 100 g lean diced ham
- ❑ Mixed green salad – as much as you want

Afternoon Snack

- ❑ A glass of water
- ❑ 8 Walnuts

Dinner

- ❑ A glass of water
- ❑ Half a grapefruit (with optional artificial sweetener)
- ❑ A glass of tomato juice
- ❑ Grilled salmon with spinach leaves*
- ❑ Ricotta cheese dessert*
  or plain or fruit low fat yoghurt
  or a small bowl of cherries or 4 dried apricots
  or either the yoghurt or fruit with sugar-free jelly
- ❑ Tea or decaffeinated coffee with optional skimmed milk and sweetener but no sugar

Menus for Day 9

Breakfast

- ❑ A glass of water
- ❑ Half a grapefruit (with optional artificial sweetener)
- ❑ Low fat fruit yoghurt
- ❑ Tea or decaffeinated coffee with optional skimmed milk and sweetener but no sugar

Morning Snack

- ❑ A glass of water
- ❑ 15 pistachio nuts

Lunch

- ❑ A glass of water
- ❑ Half a grapefruit (with optional artificial sweetener)
- ❑ 120 g grilled turkey breast
- ❑ Mixed green salad – as much as you can manage

Afternoon Snack

- ❑ A glass of water
- ❑ A bowl of cherries

Dinner

- ❑ A glass of water
- ❑ Half a grapefruit (with optional artificial sweetener)
- ❑ A glass of tomato juice
- ❑ Mexican beef stir fry* accompanied by mixed green salad
- ❑ Ricotta cheese dessert*
  or plain or fruit low fat yoghurt
  or a small bowl of cherries or 4 dried apricots
  or either the yoghurt or fruit with sugar-free jelly
- ❑ Tea or decaffeinated coffee with optional skimmed milk and sweetener but no sugar

Menus for Day 10

Breakfast

- ❑ A glass of water
- ❑ Half a grapefruit (with optional artificial sweetener)
- ❑ 2 scrambled eggs with 2 rashers of grilled lean back bacon
- ❑ Tea or decaffeinated coffee with optional skimmed milk and sweetener but no sugar

Morning Snack

- ❑ A glass of water
- ❑ Celery stick stuffed with any low fat cheese such as cottage cheese, Laughing Cow light cheese

Lunch

- ❑ A glass of water
- ❑ Half a grapefruit (with optional artificial sweetener)
- ❑ 100 g white tuna fish – in brine or water only
- ❑ Mixed green salad – as much as you can manage

Afternoon Snack

- ❑ A glass of water
- ❑ 5 Brazil nuts

Dinner

- ❑ A glass of water
- ❑ Half a grapefruit (with optional artificial sweetener)
- ❑ A glass of tomato juice
- ❑ Fillet of plaice* accompanied by broccoli spears
- ❑ Ricotta cheese dessert*
  or plain or fruit low fat yoghurt
  or a small bowl of cherries or 4 dried apricots
  or either the yoghurt or fruit with sugar-free jelly
- ❑ Tea or decaffeinated coffee with optional skimmed milk and sweetener but no sugar

Menus for Day 11

Breakfast

- ❑ A glass of water
- ❑ Half a grapefruit (with optional artificial sweetener)
- ❑ 2 eggs – poached in water, with a dash of vinegar, with 2 rashers of grilled lean back bacon
- ❑ Tea or decaffeinated coffee with optional skimmed milk and sweetener but no sugar

Morning Snack

- ❑ A glass of water
- ❑ 4 dried apricots

Lunch

- ❑ A glass of water
- ❑ Half a grapefruit (with optional artificial sweetener)
- ❑ Tomato soup*
- ❑ Low fat fruit yoghurt

Afternoon Snack

- ❑ A glass of water
- ❑ 8 cashew nuts

Dinner

- ❑ A glass of water
- ❑ Half a grapefruit (with optional artificial sweetener)
- ❑ A glass of tomato juice
- ❑ Breast of chicken with peanut butter* accompanied by greens
- ❑ Ricotta cheese dessert*
  or plain or fruit low fat yoghurt
  or a small bowl of cherries or 4 dried apricots
  or either the yoghurt or fruit with sugar-free jelly
- ❑ Tea or decaffeinated coffee with optional skimmed milk and sweetener but no sugar

Menus for Day 12

Breakfast

- ❑ A glass of water
- ❑ Half a grapefruit (with optional artificial sweetener)
- ❑ Low fat fruit yoghurt
- ❑ Tea or decaffeinated coffee with optional skimmed milk and sweetener but no sugar

Morning Snack

- ❑ A glass of water
- ❑ Celery stick stuffed with any low fat cheese such as cottage cheese, Laughing Cow light cheese

Lunch

- ❑ A glass of water
- ❑ Half a grapefruit (with optional artificial sweetener)
- ❑ 75 g lean diced ham
- ❑ Mixed green salad – as much as you can manage

Afternoon Snack

- ❑ A glass of water
- ❑ 10 peanuts, unsalted

Dinner

- ❑ A glass of water
- ❑ Half a grapefruit (with optional artificial sweetener)
- ❑ A glass of tomato juice
- ❑ Breast of turkey with courgettes*
- ❑ Ricotta cheese dessert*
  or plain or fruit low fat yoghurt
  or a small bowl of cherries or 4 dried apricots
  or either the yoghurt or fruit with sugar-free jelly
- ❑ Tea or decaffeinated coffee with optional skimmed milk and sweetener but no sugar

Menus for Day 13

Breakfast

- ❑ A glass of water
- ❑ Half a grapefruit (with optional artificial sweetener)
- ❑ 2 scrambled eggs with 2 rashers of grilled lean back bacon
- ❑ Tea or decaffeinated coffee with optional skimmed milk and sweetener but no sugar

Morning Snack

- ❑ A glass of water
- ❑ 15 pistachio nuts

Lunch

- ❑ A glass of water
- ❑ Half a grapefruit (with optional artificial sweetener)
- ❑ 120 g grilled turkey breast
- ❑ Mixed green salad – as much as you can manage

Afternoon Snack

- ❑ A glass of water
- ❑ A bowl of cherries

Dinner

- ❑ A glass of water
- ❑ Half a grapefruit (with optional artificial sweetener)
- ❑ A glass of tomato juice
- ❑ King prawn special with rocket and garlic dressing* accompanied by asparagus
- ❑ Ricotta cheese dessert*
  or plain or fruit low fat yoghurt
  or a small bowl of cherries or 4 dried apricots
  or either the yoghurt or fruit with sugar-free jelly
- ❑ Tea or decaffeinated coffee with optional skimmed milk and sweetener but no sugar

Menus for Day 14

Breakfast

- ❑ A glass of water
- ❑ Half a grapefruit (with optional artificial sweetener)
- ❑ Low fat plain yoghurt
- ❑ Tea or decaffeinated coffee with optional skimmed milk and sweetener but no sugar

Morning Snack

- ❑ A glass of water
- ❑ Celery stick stuffed with any low fat cheese such as cottage cheese, Laughing Cow light cheese

Lunch

- ❑ A glass of water
- ❑ Half a grapefruit (with optional artificial sweetener)
- ❑ Lentil soup*
- ❑ Low fat fruit yoghurt

Afternoon Snack

- ❑ A glass of water
- ❑ 8 walnuts

Dinner

- ❑ A glass of water
- ❑ Half a grapefruit (with optional artificial sweetener)
- ❑ A glass of tomato juice
- ❑ Curried pork medallions accompanied by green beans
- ❑ Ricotta cheese dessert*
  or plain or fruit low fat yoghurt
  or a small bowl of cherries or 4 dried apricots
  or either the yoghurt or fruit with sugar-free jelly
- ❑ Tea or decaffeinated coffee with optional skimmed milk and sweetener but no sugar

Chapter 15

Orientation Phase Recipes

Gazpacho

Serves 4

- ❑ 450 g (1 lb) tomatoes (peeled)
- ❑ 85 ml (3 oz) beef stock
- ❑ ½ pepper (green or red)
- ❑ 15 ml (1 tbsp) wine vinegar
- ❑ 1 courgette
- ❑ pinch of salt
- ❑ 1 cucumber
- ❑ ground black pepper
- ❑ 2 spring onions (peeled)
- ❑ 2 tspns chopped basil, chives, marjoram or thyme

Halve the tomatoes and remove the seeds. Chop the vegetables and place all the ingredients in a liquidiser or food processor and blend until the soup is perfectly smooth.

Serve well chilled (with two or three ice cubes floating in it if you like).

Tomato Soup

Serves 6

- ❑ 1 large onion
- ❑ 1 clove garlic
- ❑ 680 g (1½ lbs) tomatoes
- ❑ 1140 ml (2 pints) chicken stock
- ❑ 15 ml (1 tbspn) olive oil

- 5 g (1 level tspn) granulated artificial sweetener (optional)
- 2.5 g (½ level tspn) dried basil
- 30ml (2 tbspns) low fat natural yoghurt
- pinch of salt
- freshly ground black pepper

Skin and chop the onion. Skin and crush the garlic. Skin and chop the tomatoes (the easy way to skin tomatoes is to pour boiling water over them in a bowl and leave for about a minute). Put the oil in a large saucepan. Gently fry the onion and garlic for 5 minutes. Add the tomatoes and cook for about 2 minutes. Stir in the stock, optional sweetener, basil, salt and pepper. Bring to the boil and simmer for 30 minutes. Liquidise the soup. Reheat in a saucepan and stir in yoghurt.

Lentil Soup (Orientation Phase Version)

Serves 6

- 225 g (8 oz) lentils
- 1 onion
- 225 g (8 oz) tinned tomatoes
- olive oil for cooking
- 2 cloves garlic (crushed)
- 2 pints stock parsley

Follow the cooking instructions on the packet of lentils that you buy. Skin and chop the onion. Heat the oil in a saucepan and fry the onion for 5 minutes. Add the remaining ingredients. Bring to the boil and simmer gently for about 1 hour (depending on the type of lentil).

Serve the soup as it is or, if you prefer, liquidise it into a smooth soup. Sprinkle with parsley and season to taste.

Lentils are an excellent source of good protein. Although they are relatively deficient in sulphur-containing amino-acids they are rich in another essential amino-acid, lysine, in which many cereals are deficient. For this reason a combination of lentils and cereal provides a complete protein that compares well with animal protein. So it is a good idea to have a slice of wholegrain or sourdough bread with this soup.

Herb Chicken

Serves 4

- 4 chicken breasts with skin and fat removed
- 20 g (4 tspn) English mustard
- fresh chopped herbs – parsley, oregano, rosemary
- freshly ground black pepper
- pinch of salt
- 5 ml (1 tspn) water

Combine the mustard, herbs and water into a paste and smother both sides of the chicken, leaving some for applying later. Place in a small, shallow grill or oven tray, and cook on a low temperature until ready.

Pork Medallion Fillets

Serves 4

- 650 g (1½ lb) pork medallion fillets
- 6 dried apricots soaked in water from the morning
- rapeseed oil for cooking
- pinch of salt
- freshly ground black pepper

Remove the apricots from the water and purée them in a blender. Place the medallions in a non-stick frying pan with a smear of rapeseed oil and cook very slowly. Heat the purée gently in a small pan and then place on top of the pork. Add seasoning to taste.

Cod Fish Grill with Broccoli

Serves 4

- 4 cod fillets
- broccoli, to your taste and need
- olive oil for cooking

- ❑ 5ml (1 tspn) fresh chopped parsley
- ❑ 5 ml (1 tspn) lemon juice
- ❑ pinch of salt

Mix the olive oil, lemon juice, parsley and salt into a paste and brush the cod. Grill under a medium heat, but do not over-cook. Steam the broccoli, but do not over-cook.

Oriental Beef Stir Fry

Serves 4

- ❑ 450 g (1 lb) rump steak cut into thin slices
- ❑ green vegetables of your choice cut into stir fry pieces
- ❑ rapeseed oil for cooking
- ❑ soya sauce, to taste

Sauté the beef in rapeseed oil, add as many vegetables as you can manage. Season with soya sauce and add water, if needed, but do not over-cook.

Veal Escalope with French Beans

Serves 4

- ❑ 450 g (1 lb) veal
- ❑ French beans – as many as you can manage
- ❑ slice of low fat cheese
- ❑ 2.5 ml (½ tspn) olive oil
- ❑ 2.5 ml (½ tspn) rapeseed oil
- ❑ 5 ml (1 tspn) (no more – this is Orientation Phase!) Marsala wine
- ❑ pinch of crushed sage
- ❑ pinch of salt
- ❑ pinch of freshly ground black pepper

Lightly heat the oils in a non-stick frying pan. Season the veal and place in the frying pan and cook very gently. When cooked, place the slice of cheese on top of the veal and serve with your French beans which have been steamed, poached or boiled, according to your taste.

Fillet of Beef Steak with Asparagus

Serves 4

- ❑ 450 g fillet beef steak
- ❑ 10 asparagus spears
- ❑ 2.5 ml (½ tspn) olive oil
- ❑ 2.5 ml (½ tspn) rapeseed oil

Smear the steak with the oils and grill gently. Steam the asparagus without over-cooking.

Serve with a green salad.

Turkey Curry

Serves 4

- ❑ 4 pieces of turkey breast
- ❑ 2 dried apricots, chopped
- ❑ rapeseed oil for cooking
- ❑ homemade curry sauce (see next page)

In a non-stick frying pan gently sauté the turkey pieces lightly in oil. Add the curry sauce and simmer gently for a further minute or two. Check the taste and correct as necessary. When cooked, add the dried apricots and stir gently, adding more water if necessary.

Serve with green beans of your choice.

Curry Sauce

- ❑ 2 onions, diced
- ❑ 2 cloves garlic, chopped
- ❑ 5 g (1 tspn) ginger – fresh, chopped, dried or powdered
- ❑ 5 g (1 tspn) cumin powder
- ❑ 5 g (1 tspn) turmeric powder
- ❑ 5 g (1 tspn) cardamom seeds

- ❑ cinnamon powder or stick
- ❑ 2 cloves
- ❑ 10 g (2 tspns) coriander powder
- ❑ 10 g (2 tspns) freshly chopped coriander
- ❑ 5 g (1 tspn) freshly chopped parsley
- ❑ 15 g (1 tbspn) chillies – fresh or dried
- ❑ small amount of ordinary curry powder
- ❑ chicken or vegetable stock or water to personal taste
- ❑ rapeseed or corn oil for cooking
- ❑ 1 carton low fat yoghurt (optional)

(Quantities of each of the above ingredients depend entirely on personal taste.)

With a small amount of rapeseed or corn oil, sauté the onions and garlic in a saucepan, then empty the contents into a colander with a dish underneath. Cover with cling film and allow to stand overnight. Do not refrigerate. Next day, three-quarter fill a saucepan with stock or water and put in all the ingredients except the onion and garlic. Boil until only half of the liquid remains, then add the onion and garlic. Put everything into a hand food blender and purée. At this stage it should show the consistency of the curry sauce. You may need to reduce-down further because it is too thin for your liking, so carry on cooking. If it is too thick for your liking, add more stock or water. Now taste the flavour and adjust it to your liking, adding ingredients to suit your family's personal taste. You may at this stage add a carton of low fat plain yoghurt. You now have a fat-free, low calorie curry sauce and your diet will allow you to enjoy as much as you wish.

Curried Pork Medallions

Serves 4

- ❑ 4 medallions of pork fillet
- ❑ 1 shallot or small diced onion
- ❑ 2 dried apricots, chopped
- ❑ rapeseed oil for cooking
- ❑ 5 g (1 tspn) curry powder
- ❑ 45 ml (3 tbspns) water
- ❑ French or runner beans – to suit your taste

In a non-stick frying pan, gently sauté the medallions with the shallot/onion and when lightly browned, add the curry powder and sauté for a further minute or two. Add some water and simmer gently. When cooked, add the dried apricots and stir gently, adding more water if necessary.

Serve with the green beans of your choice.

Grilled Salmon with Spinach Leaves

Serves 4

- ❑ 4 medium-sized salmon fillets or steaks
- ❑ olive oil for cooking
- ❑ (20 ml) 4 tspn lemon juice
- ❑ pinch of fresh or dried dill
- ❑ pinch of crushed peppercorn
- ❑ pinch of salt
- ❑ a bunch of spinach leaves according to taste

Combine the oils and seasoning into a smooth paste and spread over the salmon. Grill gently, being careful not to over-cook. Cook the spinach gently with only the water that clings to the leaves and turn occasionally. Bring to the boil and then simmer until soft. Drain the spinach and serve with the salmon.

Mexican Beef Stir Fry

Serves 4

- ❑ 450 g (1 lb) rump steak, cut into thin slices
- ❑ 1 large or 2 small courgettes, cut into strips
- ❑ 10 strips of green pimentos
- ❑ 1 small onion, sliced
- ❑ a pinch of dried chilli peppers to taste
- ❑ pinch of fresh or dried parsley
- ❑ pinched of crushed peppercorns
- ❑ pinch of salt
- ❑ 10 ml (2 tspns) water

Using a non-stick frying pan, sauté the beef lightly, then add the cut vegetables and some water, stirring all the time. Add the chilli according to your taste and, if required, add more water stirring gently.

Serve with a bowl of mixed green salad.

Fillet of Plaice with Broccoli Spears

Serves 4

- ❑ 4 fillets of plaice
- ❑ broccoli spears to your need
- ❑ olive oil for cooking
- ❑ 5 g (1 tspn) English mustard
- ❑ pinch of fresh or dried parsley
- ❑ pinch of ground peppercorn

Put the plaice on a baking tray. Combine the herbs with the olive oil to make a paste and smear evenly over the fish. Grill gently until cooked. Steam or poach or boil the broccoli, drain and serve with the fish.

Breast of Chicken with Peanut Butter and Greens

Serves 4

- ❑ 4 chicken breasts with skin and fat removed
- ❑ 20 g (4 tspn) peanut butter
- ❑ 10 g (2 tspns) fresh or dried parsley
- ❑ fresh or dried chilli peppers, to taste (optional)
- ❑ greens – as many as you can manage

Combine the peanut butter and herbs into a paste and smear all over the chicken breast. Cook in a pre-heated oven at medium temperature for 15–20 minutes. Steam or poach or boil the greens, drain and serve with the chicken. A mixture of olive oil and lemon juice makes a tasty dressing if required.

Breast of Turkey with Courgettes

Serves 4

- 4 slices of turkey breast
- 30 ml (2 tbspns) low fat plain yoghurt
- pinch of ground cumin
- pinch of ginger powder
- pinch of cardamom
- pinch of ground coriander
- pinch of ground peppercorn
- pinch of salt
- ½ clove of chopped garlic
- courgettes to your need

Gently press each turkey piece into a thick escalope. Combine all the herbs with the yoghurt into a paste and coat the turkey pieces fully. Place on an oven tray and cook in a pre-heated oven at medium temperature for 10–15 minutes. Steam or poach or boil the courgettes whole, drain and serve with the turkey.

King Prawn Special with Rocket and Garlic Dressing and Asparagus

Serves 2

- 10 king prawns
- a bunch of rocket leaves
- 5 ml (1 tspn) rapeseed oil or corn oil
- 1 garlic clove, chopped
- pinch of ground peppercorn
- pinch of salt
- 10 asparagus spears

Poach or steam the prawns depending on size, but do not over-cook. Put the rocket leaves in a food blender and mix with the oil, garlic, salt and pepper, blending into a purée; water may be added if required. Steam the asparagus spears, drain and serve with the king prawns.

Grilled Tomato and Feta Cheese Salad

Serves 4

- ❑ 2 tomatoes, with skin removed and quartered and sliced into thick chunks
- ❑ 15 g (1 oz) feta cheese, sliced
- ❑ olive oil to taste
- ❑ pinch of oregano
- ❑ ground peppercorn

Using a sheet of foil, place one layer of tomato in a circle and, in the centre of this circle another layer of tomato. Evenly arrange the feta on top, but not too close together. Preheat the grill to full power, place the meal underneath and allow the feta to become golden brown. Slide portions onto individual plates, sprinkling olive oil, oregano and pepper on top.

This tasty dish is vegetarian and it can be used either as a starter or main meal. This recipe is simple, but divine! You are in the Mediterranean!

Ricotta Dessert

- ❑ 100 g (4 oz) low fat ricotta cheese
- ❑ 5 g (1 tspn) granulated artificial sweetener
- ❑ 2.5 ml (½ tspn) vanilla extract

Mix the ingredients together and place in a fridge until chilled. Serve with a sprinkling of toasted almonds or mini chocolate chips.

Two alternative dinner recipes:

Shepherd's Pie

- ❑ 450 g (1 lb) lean minced beef
- ❑ 20 courgettes
- ❑ 2 onions, diced
- ❑ rapeseed oil or corn oil for cooking
- ❑ 2 bay leaves
- ❑ 5 g (1 tspn) parsley

- ❑ Worcestershire sauce to taste
- ❑ pinch of salt
- ❑ freshly ground black pepper

Heat the oil in a non-stick saucepan, adding the onions until light brown. Add the lean minced beef and the herbs, salt and pepper to taste. When brown, with no liquid left in the saucepan, place in an oven tray and sprinkle with the sauce. Wash and cut the courgettes into chunks and steam or boil until moderately soft, then drain well. Further crush the courgettes with a fork, season to taste and spread over the tray of minced beef. Bake in a moderate, pre-heated oven for 25–30 minutes, then serve with chopped parsley to add colour and taste.

This recipe can be served with an additional vegetable of your choice. Remember to season to your liking: seasoning has no GI or fats!

Fish Curry

Serves 2

- ❑ 2 cod fish, cut into strips
- ❑ homemade curry sauce

Place the strips of cod fish evenly in an oven tray or casserole dish and cover with homemade curry sauce (see recipe in this book). Cook until tender.

Serve with steamed or boiled basmati or wild rice.

Chapter 16

Continuation Phase

This is the part for everyone. Whether you are someone who has just finished the Orientation Phase or someone else who doesn't need to lose weight but simply wants to follow a healthy diet, this is for you. This is because on the *Lose Weight Now And Forever Diet* there is no need for anyone to limit portion size or to count calories or to count grams of carbohydrates. You simply eat until you are no longer hungry. But for those who want to shed more weight there are a few little 'tweaks'.

Tweak 1: Grapefruit.

We have already looked at this in detail in Chapter 13. A brief recap: recent research has shown that eating half a grapefruit before each main meal reduces the rise in blood sugar and keeps insulin levels low. This means that we feel less hungry because high levels of insulin cause hunger. High levels of insulin also stimulate the liver to manufacture fat that increases body weight and causes coronary heart disease.

So if you still have weight to lose – and even if you haven't – grapefruit is almost a magical food. The reason that it is also good for those who don't need to lose weight is that, by keeping insulin levels low, grapefruit lowers the risk of heart disease and type 2 diabetes.

So try to eat half a grapefruit before each meal. (But please see the warning about grapefruit interactions at the end of this book.)

Tweak 2: Portion sizes

A low GI diet satisfies hunger more quickly than other diets. So to maintain weight you don't normally need to concern yourself with portion size or calories: you eat more or less as much as you like of the right kinds of food until you stop feeling hungry.

But be careful! I said above: *until you stop feeling hungry*. There is a difference between hunger and craving. So much of the excess food that we eat happens not because we are still hungry but because we crave that food. The huge portion of roast beef, the extra roast potatoes, the desserts – eating these has little to do with hunger. So we need to become more aware of hunger and to be able to distinguish it from craving.

Another way of reducing the amount of food we eat is not to start out each meal feeling ravenous. Feeling ravenous means that our blood sugar is low. A light snack between meals or shortly before a meal works wonders for this. Good examples are a slice of low fat cheese, a piece of fruit or carrot, or a few nuts. It takes much less food to prevent a low blood sugar than it does to correct it.

The Continuation Phase is for life. Initially follow the recipe suggestions in this book. Then, as you become more experienced and familiar with low GI foods and cooking methods, you can start to devise your own menus.

If, for any reason, you find that your diet has slipped and that your weight has increased again – no-one is perfect – go back to the Orientation Phase for a couple of weeks, and then return to Continuation.

Chapter 17

Continuation Phase Menus

Menus for Day 1 – Monday

Breakfast

- ❑ A glass of water
- ❑ Half a grapefruit (with optional artificial sweetener)
- ❑ Tea or decaffeinated coffee with optional skimmed or soya milk and sweetener but no sugar

Choice of the following:

- ❑ An approved breakfast cereal – look up the Guidelines
- ❑ Low fat plain yoghurt
- ❑ Low fat fruit yoghurt
- ❑ Scrambled egg on wholegrain toast
- ❑ Poached egg with lean-grilled ham, tomato and grilled mushrooms
- ❑ Two boiled eggs with wholegrain toast 'soldiers'

Morning Snack

- ❑ A glass of water

Choice of:

- ❑ Vegetable sticks (eg carrots, celery, cauliflower)
- ❑ Celery stick with low fat cheese eg cottage, Laughing Cow
- ❑ Celery stick or apple with 5 g (1 tspn) peanut butter
- ❑ Low fat sugar-free yoghurt
- ❑ Nuts (within the daily permitted quantity)
- ❑ Tea or decaffeinated coffee with optional skimmed or soya milk and sweetener but no sugar

Lunch

- ❑ A glass of water
- ❑ Half a grapefruit (with optional artificial sweetener)
- ❑ Stuffed Peppers*

Afternoon Snack

- ❑ A glass of water

Choice of:

- ❑ Vegetable sticks (eg carrots, celery, cauliflower)
- ❑ Celery stick with low fat cheese eg cottage, Laughing Cow
- ❑ Celery stick or apple with 5 g (1 tspn) peanut butter
- ❑ Low fat sugar-free yoghurt

- ❑ Nuts (within the daily permitted quantity)
- ❑ Tea or decaffeinated coffee with optional skimmed or soya milk and sweetener but no sugar

Dinner

- ❑ A glass of water
- ❑ Half a grapefruit (with optional artificial sweetener)
- ❑ Lemon Chicken*
- ❑ Fruit Pavlova or Slimmers' Meringue*

Menus for Day 2 – Tuesday

Breakfast

- ❑ A glass of water
- ❑ Half a grapefruit (with optional artificial sweetener)
- ❑ Tea or decaffeinated coffee with optional skimmed or soya milk and sweetener but no sugar

Choice of the following:

- ❑ An approved breakfast cereal – look up the Guidelines
- ❑ Low fat plain yoghurt
- ❑ Low fat fruit yoghurt
- ❑ Scrambled egg on wholegrain toast
- ❑ Poached egg with lean-grilled ham, tomato and grilled mushrooms
- ❑ Two boiled eggs with wholegrain toast 'soldiers'

Morning Snack

- ❑ A glass of water

Choice of:

- ❑ Vegetable sticks (eg carrots, celery, cauliflower)
- ❑ Celery stick with low fat cheese eg cottage, Laughing Cow
- ❑ Celery stick or apple with 5 g (1 tspn) peanut butter
- ❑ Low fat sugar-free yoghurt
- ❑ Nuts (within the daily permitted quantity)
- ❑ Tea or decaffeinated coffee with optional skimmed or soya milk and sweetener but no sugar

Lunch

- ❑ A glass of water
- ❑ Half a grapefruit (with optional artificial sweetener)
- ❑ Ham and low fat (eg Laughing Cow) cheese sandwich, using wholegrain or sourdough bread
- ❑ You may add salad ingredients if you wish

Afternoon Snack

- ❑ A glass of water
- ❑ Choice of:
- ❑ Vegetable sticks (eg carrots, celery, cauliflower)
- ❑ Celery stick with low fat cheese eg cottage, Laughing Cow
- ❑ Celery stick or apple with 5 g (1 tspn) peanut butter
- ❑ Low fat sugar-free yoghurt
- ❑ Nuts (within the daily permitted quantity)
- ❑ Tea or decaffeinated coffee with optional skimmed or soya milk and sweetener but no sugar

Dinner

- ❑ A glass of water
- ❑ Half a grapefruit (with optional artificial sweetener)
- ❑ Spicey Haddock Parcels*
- ❑ Peach Melba*

Menus for Day 3 – Wednesday

Breakfast

- ❑ A glass of water
- ❑ Half a grapefruit (with optional artificial sweetener)
- ❑ Tea or decaffeinated coffee with optional skimmed or soya milk and sweetener but no sugar

Choice of the following:

- ❑ An approved breakfast cereal – look up the Guidelines
- ❑ Low fat plain yoghurt
- ❑ Low fat fruit yoghurt
- ❑ Scrambled egg on wholegrain toast
- ❑ Poached egg with lean-grilled ham, tomato and grilled mushrooms
- ❑ Two boiled eggs with wholegrain toast 'soldiers'

Morning Snack

- ❑ A glass of water

Choice of:

- ❑ Vegetable sticks (eg carrots, celery, cauliflower)
- ❑ Celery stick with low fat cheese eg cottage, Laughing Cow
- ❑ Celery stick or apple with 5 g (1 tspn) peanut butter
- ❑ Low fat sugar-free yoghurt
- ❑ Nuts (within the daily permitted quantity)
- ❑ Tea or decaffeinated coffee with optional skimmed or soya milk and sweetener but no sugar

Lunch

- ❑ A glass of water
- ❑ Half a grapefruit (with optional artificial sweetener)
- ❑ Pasta and Chicken Salad*

Afternoon Snack

- ❑ A glass of water

Choice of:

- ❑ Vegetable sticks (eg carrots, celery, cauliflower)
- ❑ Celery stick with low fat cheese eg cottage, Laughing Cow
- ❑ Celery stick or apple with 5 g (1 tspn) peanut butter
- ❑ Low fat sugar-free yoghurt
- ❑ Nuts (within the daily permitted quantity)
- ❑ Tea or decaffeinated coffee with optional skimmed or soya milk and sweetener but no sugar

Dinner

- ❑ A glass of water
- ❑ Half a grapefruit (with optional artificial sweetener)
- ❑ Lamb Curry*
- ❑ Apple Mousse*

Menus for Day 4 – Thursday

Breakfast

- ❑ A glass of water
- ❑ Half a grapefruit (with optional artificial sweetener)
- ❑ Tea or decaffeinated coffee with optional skimmed or soya milk and sweetener but no sugar

Choice of the following:

- ❑ An approved breakfast cereal – look up the Guidelines
- ❑ Low fat plain yoghurt
- ❑ Low fat fruit yoghurt
- ❑ Scrambled egg on wholegrain toast
- ❑ Poached egg with lean-grilled ham, tomato and grilled mushrooms
- ❑ Two boiled eggs with wholegrain toast 'soldiers'

Morning Snack

- ❑ A glass of water
- ❑ Choice of:
- ❑ Vegetable sticks (eg carrots, celery, cauliflower)
- ❑ Celery stick with low fat cheese eg cottage, Laughing Cow
- ❑ Celery stick or apple with 5 g (1 tspn) peanut butter
- ❑ Low fat sugar-free yoghurt
- ❑ Nuts (within the daily permitted quantity)
- ❑ Tea or decaffeinated coffee with optional skimmed or soya milk and sweetener but no sugar

Lunch

- ❑ A glass of water
- ❑ Half a grapefruit (with optional artificial sweetener)
- ❑ Beef Kebabs*

Afternoon Snack

- ❑ A glass of water

Choice of:

- ❑ Vegetable sticks (eg carrots, celery, cauliflower)
- ❑ Celery stick with low fat cheese eg cottage, Laughing Cow
- ❑ Celery stick or apple with 5 g (1 tspn) peanut butter
- ❑ Low fat sugar-free yoghurt
- ❑ Nuts (within the daily permitted quantity)
- ❑ Tea or decaffeinated coffee with optional skimmed or soya milk and sweetener but no sugar

Dinner

- ❑ A glass of water
- ❑ Half a grapefruit (with optional artificial sweetener)
- ❑ Chicken Rosemary*
- ❑ Orange Sorbet*

Menus for Day 5 – Friday

Breakfast

- ❑ A glass of water
- ❑ Half a grapefruit (with optional artificial sweetener)
- ❑ Tea or decaffeinated coffee with optional skimmed or soya milk and sweetener but no sugar

Choice of the following:

- ❑ An approved breakfast cereal – look up the Guidelines
- ❑ Low fat plain yoghurt
- ❑ Low fat fruit yoghurt
- ❑ Scrambled egg on wholegrain toast
- ❑ Poached egg with lean-grilled ham, tomato and grilled mushrooms
- ❑ Two boiled eggs with wholegrain toast 'soldiers'

Morning Snack

- ❑ A glass of water

Choice of:

- ❑ Vegetable sticks (eg carrots, celery, cauliflower)
- ❑ Celery stick with low fat cheese eg cottage, Laughing Cow
- ❑ Celery stick or apple with 5 g (1 tspn) peanut butter
- ❑ Low fat sugar-free yoghurt
- ❑ Nuts (within the daily permitted quantity)
- ❑ Tea or decaffeinated coffee with optional skimmed or soya milk and sweetener but no sugar

Lunch

- ❑ A glass of water
- ❑ Half a grapefruit (with optional artificial sweetener)
- ❑ Tuna and Pasta Salad*

Afternoon Snack

- ❑ A glass of water

Choice of:

- ❑ Vegetable sticks (eg carrots, celery, cauliflower)
- ❑ Celery stick with low fat cheese eg cottage, Laughing Cow
- ❑ Celery stick or apple with 5 g (1 tspn) peanut butter
- ❑ Low fat sugar-free yoghurt
- ❑ Nuts (within the daily permitted quantity)
- ❑ Tea or decaffeinated coffee with optional skimmed or soya milk and sweetener but no sugar

Dinner

- ❑ A glass of water
- ❑ Half a grapefruit (with optional artificial sweetener)
- ❑ Veal in Breadcrumbs*
- ❑ Apple and Lemon Compote*

Menus for Day 6 – Saturday

Breakfast

- ❑ A glass of water
- ❑ Half a grapefruit (with optional artificial sweetener)
- ❑ Tea or decaffeinated coffee with optional skimmed or soya milk and sweetener but no sugar

Choice of the following:

- ❑ An approved breakfast cereal – look up the Guidelines
- ❑ Low fat plain yoghurt
- ❑ Low fat fruit yoghurt
- ❑ Scrambled egg on wholegrain toast
- ❑ Poached egg with lean-grilled ham, tomato and grilled mushrooms
- ❑ Two boiled eggs with wholegrain toast 'soldiers'

Morning Snack

- ❑ A glass of water

Choice of:

- ❑ Vegetable sticks (eg carrots, celery, cauliflower)
- ❑ Celery stick with low fat cheese eg cottage, Laughing Cow
- ❑ Celery stick or apple with 5 g (1 tspn) peanut butter
- ❑ Low fat sugar-free yoghurt
- ❑ Nuts (within the daily permitted quantity)
- ❑ Tea or decaffeinated coffee with optional skimmed or soya milk and sweetener but no sugar

Lunch

- ❑ A glass of water
- ❑ Half a grapefruit (with optional artificial sweetener)
- ❑ Tuna Salad* with Mushroom Marinade*

Afternoon Snack

- ❑ A glass of water

Choice of:

- ❑ Vegetable sticks (eg carrots, celery, cauliflower)
- ❑ Celery stick with low fat cheese eg cottage, Laughing Cow
- ❑ Celery stick or apple with 5 g (1 tspn) peanut butter
- ❑ Low fat sugar-free yoghurt
- ❑ Nuts (within the daily permitted quantity)
- ❑ Tea or decaffeinated coffee with optional skimmed or soya milk and sweetener but no sugar

Dinner

- ❑ A glass of water
- ❑ Half a grapefruit (with optional artificial sweetener)
- ❑ Chicken with Basmati Rice*
- ❑ Raspberry Sorbet*

Menus for Day 7 – Sunday

Breakfast

- ❑ A glass of water
- ❑ Half a grapefruit (with optional artificial sweetener)
- ❑ Tea or decaffeinated coffee with optional skimmed or soya milk and sweetener but no sugar

Choice of the following:

- ❑ An approved breakfast cereal – look up the Guidelines
- ❑ Low fat plain yoghurt
- ❑ Low fat fruit yoghurt
- ❑ Scrambled egg on wholegrain toast
- ❑ Poached egg with lean-grilled ham, tomato and grilled mushrooms
- ❑ Two boiled eggs with wholegrain toast 'soldiers'

Morning Snack

- ❑ A glass of water

Choice of:

- ❑ Vegetable sticks (eg carrots, celery, cauliflower)
- ❑ Celery stick with low fat cheese eg cottage, Laughing Cow
- ❑ Celery stick or apple with 5 g (1 tspn) peanut butter
- ❑ Low fat sugar-free yoghurt
- ❑ Nuts (within the daily permitted quantity)
- ❑ Tea or decaffeinated coffee with optional skimmed or soya milk and sweetener but no sugar

Lunch

- ❑ A glass of water
- ❑ Half a grapefruit (with optional artificial sweetener)
- ❑ Mushroom and Onion Bake*

Afternoon Snack

- ❑ A glass of water

Choice of:

- ❑ Vegetable sticks (eg carrots, celery, cauliflower)
- ❑ Celery stick with low fat cheese eg cottage, Laughing Cow
- ❑ Celery stick or apple with 5 g (1 tspn) peanut butter
- ❑ Low fat sugar-free yoghurt
- ❑ Nuts (within the daily permitted quantity)
- ❑ Tea or decaffeinated coffee with optional skimmed or soya milk and sweetener but no sugar

Dinner

- ❑ A glass of water
- ❑ Half a grapefruit (with optional artificial sweetener)
- ❑ Roast Lamb with Garlic*
- ❑ Chocolate Soufflé*

Menus for Day 8 – Monday

Breakfast

- ❑ A glass of water
- ❑ Half a grapefruit (with optional artificial sweetener)
- ❑ Tea or decaffeinated coffee with optional skimmed or soya milk and sweetener but no sugar

Choice of the following:

- ❑ An approved breakfast cereal – look up the Guidelines
- ❑ Low fat plain yoghurt
- ❑ Low fat fruit yoghurt
- ❑ Scrambled egg on wholegrain toast
- ❑ Poached egg with lean-grilled ham, tomato and grilled mushrooms
- ❑ Two boiled eggs with wholegrain toast 'soldiers'

Morning Snack

- ❑ A glass of water

Choice of:

- ❑ Vegetable sticks (eg carrots, celery, cauliflower)
- ❑ Celery stick with low fat cheese eg cottage, Laughing Cow
- ❑ Celery stick or apple with 5 g (1 tspn) peanut butter
- ❑ Low fat sugar-free yoghurt
- ❑ Nuts (within the daily permitted quantity)
- ❑ Tea or decaffeinated coffee with optional skimmed or soya milk and sweetener but no sugar

Lunch

- ❑ A glass of water
- ❑ Half a grapefruit (with optional artificial sweetener)
- ❑ Lamb Kebab*

Afternoon Snack

- ❑ A glass of water

Choice of:

- ❑ Vegetable sticks (eg carrots, celery, cauliflower)
- ❑ Celery stick with low fat cheese eg cottage, Laughing Cow
- ❑ Celery stick or apple with 5 g (1 tspn) peanut butter
- ❑ Low fat sugar-free yoghurt
- ❑ Nuts (within the daily permitted quantity)
- ❑ Tea or decaffeinated coffee with optional skimmed or soya milk and sweetener but no sugar

Dinner

- ❑ A glass of water
- ❑ Half a grapefruit (with optional artificial sweetener)
- ❑ Chicken Casserole* with Basmati or Wild Rice

Menus for Day 9 – Tuesday

Breakfast

- ❑ A glass of water
- ❑ Half a grapefruit (with optional artificial sweetener)
- ❑ Tea or decaffeinated coffee with optional skimmed or soya milk and sweetener but no sugar

  Choice of the following:
- ❑ An approved breakfast cereal – look up the Guidelines
- ❑ Low fat plain yoghurt
- ❑ Low fat fruit yoghurt
- ❑ Scrambled egg on wholegrain toast
- ❑ Poached egg with lean-grilled ham, tomato and grilled mushrooms
- ❑ Two boiled eggs with wholegrain toast 'soldiers'

Morning Snack

- ❑ A glass of water

  Choice of:
- ❑ Vegetable sticks (eg carrots, celery, cauliflower)
- ❑ Celery stick with low fat cheese eg cottage, Laughing Cow
- ❑ Celery stick or apple with 5 g (1 tspn) peanut butter
- ❑ Low fat sugar-free yoghurt
- ❑ Nuts (within the daily permitted quantity)
- ❑ Tea or decaffeinated coffee with optional skimmed or soya milk and sweetener but no sugar

Lunch

- ❑ A glass of water
- ❑ Half a grapefruit (with optional artificial sweetener)
- ❑ Carrot and Onion Soup*
- ❑ Red Cabbage Crunchy Salad*

Afternoon Snack

- ❑ A glass of water

  Choice of:
- ❑ Vegetable sticks (eg carrots, celery, cauliflower)
- ❑ Celery stick with low fat cheese eg cottage, Laughing Cow
- ❑ Celery stick or apple with 5 g (1 tspn) peanut butter
- ❑ Low fat sugar-free yoghurt
- ❑ Nuts (within the daily permitted quantity)
- ❑ Tea or decaffeinated coffee with optional skimmed or soya milk and sweetener but no sugar

Dinner

- ❑ A glass of water
- ❑ Half a grapefruit (with optional artificial sweetener)
- ❑ Cod with Cucumber*
- ❑ Orange and Rhubarb*

Menus for Day 10 – Wednesday

Breakfast

- ❑ A glass of water
- ❑ Half a grapefruit (with optional artificial sweetener)
- ❑ Tea or decaffeinated coffee with optional skimmed or soya milk and sweetener but no sugar

Choice of the following:

- ❑ An approved breakfast cereal – look up the Guidelines
- ❑ Low fat plain yoghurt
- ❑ Low fat fruit yoghurt
- ❑ Scrambled egg on wholegrain toast
- ❑ Poached egg with lean-grilled ham, tomato and grilled mushrooms
- ❑ Two boiled eggs with wholegrain toast 'soldiers'

Morning Snack

- ❑ A glass of water

Choice of:

- ❑ Vegetable sticks (eg carrots, celery, cauliflower)
- ❑ Celery stick with low fat cheese eg cottage, Laughing Cow
- ❑ Celery stick or apple with 5 g (1 tspn) peanut butter
- ❑ Low fat sugar-free yoghurt
- ❑ Nuts (within the daily permitted quantity)
- ❑ Tea or decaffeinated coffee with optional skimmed or soya milk and sweetener but no sugar

Lunch

- ❑ A glass of water
- ❑ Half a grapefruit (with optional artificial sweetener)
- ❑ Vegetable Curry*

Afternoon Snack

- ❑ A glass of water

Choice of:

- ❑ Vegetable sticks (eg carrots, celery, cauliflower)
- ❑ Celery stick with low fat cheese eg cottage, Laughing Cow
- ❑ Celery stick or apple with 5 g (1 tspn) peanut butter
- ❑ Low fat sugar-free yoghurt
- ❑ Nuts (within the daily permitted quantity)
- ❑ Tea or decaffeinated coffee with optional skimmed or soya milk and sweetener but no sugar

Dinner

- ❑ A glass of water
- ❑ Half a grapefruit (with optional artificial sweetener)
- ❑ Chicken Peppery Pasta*
- ❑ Plum and Pear Compote*

Menus for Day 11 – Thursday

Breakfast

- ❑ A glass of water
- ❑ Half a grapefruit (with optional artificial sweetener)
- ❑ Tea or decaffeinated coffee with optional skimmed or soya milk and sweetener but no sugar

Choice of the following:

- ❑ An approved breakfast cereal – look up the Guidelines
- ❑ Low fat plain yoghurt
- ❑ Low fat fruit yoghurt
- ❑ Scrambled egg on wholegrain toast
- ❑ Poached egg with lean-grilled ham, tomato and grilled mushrooms
- ❑ Two boiled eggs with wholegrain toast 'soldiers'

Morning Snack

- ❑ A glass of water

Choice of:

- ❑ Vegetable sticks (eg carrots, celery, cauliflower)
- ❑ Celery stick with low fat cheese eg cottage, Laughing Cow
- ❑ Celery stick or apple with 5 g (1 tspn) peanut butter
- ❑ Low fat sugar-free yoghurt
- ❑ Nuts (within the daily permitted quantity)
- ❑ Tea or decaffeinated coffee with optional skimmed or soya milk and sweetener but no sugar

Lunch

- ❑ A glass of water
- ❑ Half a grapefruit (with optional artificial sweetener)
- ❑ Lentil Soup*
- ❑ Celery, Radish and Green Pepper Salad*

Afternoon Snack

- ❑ A glass of water

Choice of:

- ❑ Vegetable sticks (eg carrots, celery, cauliflower)
- ❑ Celery stick with low fat cheese eg cottage, Laughing Cow
- ❑ Celery stick or apple with 5 g (1 tspn) peanut butter
- ❑ Low fat sugar-free yoghurt
- ❑ Nuts (within the daily permitted quantity)
- ❑ Tea or decaffeinated coffee with optional skimmed or soya milk and sweetener but no sugar

Dinner

- ❑ A glass of water
- ❑ Half a grapefruit (with optional artificial sweetener)
- ❑ Grilled Sole with Grapes*
- ❑ Apple and Blackberry Compote*

Menus for Day 12 – Friday

Breakfast

- ❑ A glass of water
- ❑ Half a grapefruit (with optional artificial sweetener)
- ❑ Tea or decaffeinated coffee with optional skimmed or soya milk and sweetener but no sugar

  Choice of the following:
- ❑ An approved breakfast cereal – look up the Guidelines
- ❑ Low fat plain yoghurt
- ❑ Low fat fruit yoghurt
- ❑ Scrambled egg on wholegrain toast
- ❑ Poached egg with lean-grilled ham, tomato and grilled mushrooms
- ❑ Two boiled eggs with wholegrain toast 'soldiers'

Morning Snack

- ❑ A glass of water

  Choice of:
- ❑ Vegetable sticks (eg carrots, celery, cauliflower)
- ❑ Celery stick with low fat cheese eg cottage, Laughing Cow
- ❑ Celery stick or apple with 5 g (1 tspn) peanut butter
- ❑ Low fat sugar-free yoghurt
- ❑ Nuts (within the daily permitted quantity)
- ❑ Tea or decaffeinated coffee with optional skimmed or soya milk and sweetener but no sugar

Lunch

- ❑ A glass of water
- ❑ Half a grapefruit (with optional artificial sweetener)
- ❑ French Onion Soup*
- ❑ Red Pepper and Beanshoot Salad*

Afternoon Snack

- ❑ A glass of water

  Choice of:
- ❑ Vegetable sticks (eg carrots, celery, cauliflower)
- ❑ Celery stick with low fat cheese eg cottage, Laughing Cow
- ❑ Celery stick or apple with 5 g (1 tspn) peanut butter
- ❑ Low fat sugar-free yoghurt
- ❑ Nuts (within the daily permitted quantity)
- ❑ Tea or decaffeinated coffee with optional skimmed or soya milk and sweetener but no sugar

Dinner

- ❑ A glass of water
- ❑ Half a grapefruit (with optional artificial sweetener)
- ❑ Chicken Curry*
- ❑ Lemon Jelly with Banana*

Menus for Day 13 – Saturday

Breakfast

- ❑ A glass of water
- ❑ Half a grapefruit (with optional artificial sweetener)
- ❑ Tea or decaffeinated coffee with optional skimmed or soya milk and sweetener but no sugar

Choice of the following:

- ❑ An approved breakfast cereal – look up the Guidelines
- ❑ Low fat plain yoghurt
- ❑ Low fat fruit yoghurt
- ❑ Scrambled egg on wholegrain toast
- ❑ Poached egg with lean-grilled ham, tomato and grilled mushrooms
- ❑ Two boiled eggs with wholegrain toast 'soldiers'

Morning Snack

- ❑ A glass of water

Choice of:

- ❑ Vegetable sticks (eg carrots, celery, cauliflower)
- ❑ Celery stick with low fat cheese eg cottage, Laughing Cow
- ❑ Celery stick or apple with 5 g (1 tspn) peanut butter
- ❑ Low fat sugar-free yoghurt
- ❑ Nuts (within the daily permitted quantity)
- ❑ Tea or decaffeinated coffee with optional skimmed or soya milk and sweetener but no sugar

Lunch

- ❑ A glass of water
- ❑ Half a grapefruit (with optional artificial sweetener)
- ❑ Chilli Bean and Frankfurter Salad*

Afternoon Snack

- ❑ A glass of water

Choice of:

- ❑ Vegetable sticks (eg carrots, celery, cauliflower)
- ❑ Celery stick with low fat cheese eg cottage, Laughing Cow
- ❑ Celery stick or apple with 5 g (1 tspn) peanut butter
- ❑ Low fat sugar-free yoghurt
- ❑ Nuts (within the daily permitted quantity)
- ❑ Tea or decaffeinated coffee with optional skimmed or soya milk and sweetener but no sugar

Dinner

- ❑ A glass of water
- ❑ Half a grapefruit (with optional artificial sweetener)
- ❑ Haddock in Parsley Sauce*
- ❑ Hot Fruit Compote*

Menus for Day 14 – Sunday

Breakfast

- ❑ A glass of water
- ❑ Half a grapefruit (with optional artificial sweetener)
- ❑ Tea or decaffeinated coffee with optional skimmed or soya milk and sweetener but no sugar

Choice of the following:

- ❑ An approved breakfast cereal – look up the Guidelines
- ❑ Low fat plain yoghurt
- ❑ Low fat fruit yoghurt
- ❑ Scrambled egg on wholegrain toast
- ❑ Poached egg with lean-grilled ham, tomato and grilled mushrooms
- ❑ Two boiled eggs with wholegrain toast 'soldiers'

Morning Snack

- ❑ A glass of water

Choice of:

- ❑ Vegetable sticks (eg carrots, celery, cauliflower)
- ❑ Celery stick with low fat cheese eg cottage, Laughing Cow
- ❑ Celery stick or apple with 5 g (1 tspn) peanut butter
- ❑ Low fat sugar-free yoghurt
- ❑ Nuts (within the daily permitted quantity)
- ❑ Tea or decaffeinated coffee with optional skimmed or soya milk and sweetener but no sugar

Lunch

- ❑ A glass of water
- ❑ Half a grapefruit (with optional artificial sweetener)
- ❑ Celery Soup*
- ❑ Cucumber Jelly*

Afternoon Snack

- ❑ A glass of water

Choice of:

- ❑ Vegetable sticks (eg carrots, celery, cauliflower)
- ❑ Celery stick with low fat cheese eg cottage, Laughing Cow
- ❑ Celery stick or apple with 5 g (1 tspn) peanut butter
- ❑ Low fat sugar-free yoghurt
- ❑ Nuts (within the daily permitted quantity)
- ❑ Tea or decaffeinated coffee with optional skimmed or soya milk and sweetener but no sugar

Dinner

- ❑ A glass of water
- ❑ Half a grapefruit (with optional artificial sweetener)
- ❑ Roast Beef with Wholemeal Yorkshire Pudding*
- ❑ Crêpes Suzette*

(Yes, you read the above correctly! This menu is a little reward for you. But you will see that the dishes are prepared in a low GI way.)

Chapter 18

Continuation Phase Recipes

Stuffed Peppers

Serves 4

- ❑ 4 green peppers
- ❑ 340 mg (12 oz) lean minced beef
- ❑ 115 g (4 oz) mushrooms
- ❑ 2 carrots
- ❑ 396 g (14 oz) tinned tomatoes
- ❑ 2 small onions
- ❑ 2 cloves garlic, crushed
- ❑ pinch mixed dried herbs
- ❑ 285 ml (½ pint) stock
- ❑ pinch of salt
- ❑ freshly ground black pepper

Fry the beef in its own fat in a non-stick pan. Meanwhile grate the carrots, chop the mushrooms, finely chop the onions, and slice the stalk off the peppers and remove the cores and seeds. Drain off the fat from the beef and add the onions, carrots, mushrooms and garlic. Cook on a low heat until the onions are soft, then add the tomatoes (but not the juice), the herbs and seasoning. Stuff the peppers with the beef and vegetable mixture, then place the peppers in a dish and pour over the juice of the tomatoes and stock. Cover and cook gently in an oven, gas mark 2, 350°F (180°C), for 45 minutes.

Lemon Chicken

Serves 4

- 4 chicken breasts
- 55 ml (4 tbspns) fresh lemon juice
- rind of one lemon (grated)
- 30 ml (2 tbspns) rapeseed or corn oil
- 2 cloves garlic (crushed)
- pinch of salt
- freshly ground black pepper

Place the chicken breasts in a greased shallow baking dish. Mix the lemon juice, rind, oil and garlic together. Lightly sprinkle the chicken pieces with a little salt and pepper. Pour the lemon mixture evenly over the chicken. Cover and bake in an oven, gas mark 4, 350°F (180°C), for 45 minutes, basting occasionally. Remove the cover and cook for a further 15 minutes to allow the chicken to brown slightly. Before serving, remove the chicken skin and sprinkle with chopped parsley.

Fruit Pavlova or Slimmers' Meringue

Serves 4

- 3 large egg whites
- 5 ml (1 tspn) cream of tartar
- 45 g (3 tbspns) skimmed milk powder
- 30 g (2 tbspns) granulated sweetener
- 1 410g (14½ oz) tin of fruit salad in unsweetened syrup
- 6 sprigs mint

Whisk the egg whites, add the cream of tartar, and continue whisking until the mixture stiffens and peaks form. Add the skimmed milk powder and sweetener, and continue whisking until peaks form again. On a sheet of non-stick paper, draw a circle round an 20 cm (8-inch) plate. Place on a baking sheet, and spread (or pipe) the mixture smoothly in the circle. Cook in a pre-heated oven, gas mark 1, 275°F (140°C), for one hour. Cool, then loosen carefully with a palette knife and place on a serving dish. Drain the fruit salad and pile on top of the meringue, and top with the sprigs of mint.

Spicey Haddock Parcels

Serves 4

- 4 170g (6 oz) haddock fillets
- 225 g (8 oz) mushrooms
- 2.5g (½ tspn) ground ginger
- 10g (2 tspns) soy sauce
- 45m (1½ tbspns) lemon juice
- 30 g (1 oz) rapeseed or corn oil
- pinch of salt
- freshly ground black pepper

Remove the skin from the fish. Take 4 pieces of foil large enough to wrap each fillet of haddock in and place a fillet on each. Slice the mushrooms. Mix together the lemon juice, ginger, soy sauce and oil. Put one-quarter of the mixture on top of each fillet and then place the mushrooms evenly on top. Season with salt and pepper and fold over the foil to make 4 parcels. Bake in the oven, gas mark 4, 350°F (180°C), for 40 minutes.

Serve with basmati rice and green salad.

Peach Melba

Serves 2

- 275 ml (½ pint) low-fat natural yoghurt
- 2.5 ml (½ tspn) liquid sweetener
- 1 egg white
- 2.5 ml (½ tspn) vanilla essence
- 55 g (2 oz) raspberries
- peach slices

Blend together the yoghurt and sweetener and chill in the freezer. Whisk the egg white. Turn the yoghurt mixture into a bowl, add the vanilla essence and egg white, and freeze until firm. Sieve the raspberries to make a smooth purée and blend together with the sweetener to taste. Scoop out the ice-cream, serve with the purée, and decorate with slices of peach.

Pasta and Chicken Salad

Serves 4

- ❑ 115 g (4 oz) wholewheat or durum wheat pasta rings or shells
- ❑ 225 g (8 oz) cooked chicken
- ❑ 2 red apples
- ❑ 2 sticks celery
- ❑ pinch of salt
- ❑ freshly ground black pepper
- ❑ 30 ml (2 tbspns) homemade low GI mayonnaise (see recipe in this book)
- ❑ 15 ml (1 tbspn) natural low-fat yoghurt

Cook the pasta *al dente* according to the instructions on the packet. Leave to cool. Remove the skin from the chicken and cut the flesh into bite-sized pieces. Core and dice the apple. Chop the celery and mix with the pasta, chicken and apple. Season. Add the mayonnaise mixed with yoghurt and evenly coat the chicken-pasta mixture. Serve on a bed of lettuce.

Lamb Curry

Serves 4

- ❑ 450 g (1 lb) lean lamb, cut into cubes
- ❑ 10 g (2 tspns) tomato purée
- ❑ 1 large tomato, diced
- ❑ fresh chopped coriander
- ❑ 15 g (1 oz) chillies – fresh or dried
- ❑ rapeseed oil or corn oil for cooking

In a large non-stick frying pan or saucepan, sauté the lamb until brown, then add the tomato purée, fresh chopped coriander and chillies, and further sauté. When ready, add homemade curry sauce (see page 80) and cook in the saucepan, or if preferred, in an oven, until the meat is tender.

Serve with steamed or boiled basmati or wild rice.

Apple Mousse

- ❑ 455 g (1 lb) cooking apples
- ❑ 30 g (2 tbspns) redcurrant jelly
- ❑ 1 egg white
- ❑ ground cinnamon
- ❑ 100 ml (1 teacup) water

Peel, slice and core the apples, and cook them until tender. Whilst the fruit is hot add the redcurrant jelly. Liquidise the apple mixture. Allow the mixture to cool. Whisk the egg white until it is stiff, and then fold into the apple mixture. Spoon the mixture into four glass bowls.

Serve chilled with a little cinnamon sprinkled on top.

Beef Kebabs

Serves 4

- ❑ 455g (1 lb) rump steak
- ❑ 2 onions
- ❑ 1 green pepper
- ❑ 1 red pepper
- ❑ 115 g (4 oz) button mushrooms
- ❑ 225 ml (8 oz) tomato juice (unsweetened)
- ❑ 2 cloves garlic, crushed
- ❑ 5 g (1 tspn) dried mixed herbs
- ❑ 15 ml (1 tbspn) soy sauce
- ❑ pinch of salt
- ❑ freshly ground black pepper

Cut all the visible fat off the steak and cut the meat into large cubes. Mix together the tomato juice, garlic, herbs, soy sauce, salt and pepper. Place the meat in a bowl, pour over the tomato juice mixture, cover with cling film, and marinade for several hours, turning the meat from time to time. Meanwhile peel the onions and cut into quarters. Slice the stalk end off the peppers, remove the cores and seeds, and cut into eight pieces.

When marinaded drain the steak. Take a skewer and thread the meat on to it, alternating with a piece of onion, a piece of pepper and a mushroom, until the skewer is nearly full. Do the same with three more skewers. Grill each skewer under a pre-heated grill, turning frequently, for 15 to 20 minutes, until the meat is well done.

These kebabs are also delicious cooked on a barbecue when they can be served with new or sweet potatoes or basmati rice.

Chicken Rosemary

Serves 4

- ❑ 4 chicken breasts, with skins removed
- ❑ 10 g (2 tspns) dried rosemary (or fresh if you have it)
- ❑ pinch of salt
- ❑ freshly ground black pepper

Rub the rosemary, salt and pepper into the chicken. Wrap the chicken pieces in foil and bake in an oven, gas mark 5, 375°F (190°C), for 1 hour. Serve with basmati rice or sweet potato and green vegetables.

Orange Sorbet

Serves 4

- ❑ 1 x 170 g (6 oz) can unsweetened orange juice
- ❑ 30 ml (2 tbspns) lemon juice
- ❑ 1 egg white
- ❑ 5 ml (1 tspn) liquid sweetener
- ❑ 285ml (½ pint) water

Mix together the orange juice, lemon juice, sweetener and water and pour into a suitable container to place in a freezer (such as an ice-cube tray or an old ice-cream tub) and freeze until just firm. Remove from the freezer and tip the mixture into a bowl and mash with a fork or potato masher until the crystals are broken down. Whisk the egg white until stiff and fold into the orange mixture. Once again pour the mixture into a container and freeze until firm.

Before serving place the mixture in a fridge for about 20 minutes to allow it to soften slightly. Serve in glass dishes and decorate with a twist of orange or sprig of mint.

Tuna and Pasta Salad

Serves 4

- ½ tin, ie 99g (3½ oz) tuna in brine
- 115 g (4 oz) wholewheat pasta tubes or shells
- 30 ml (2 tbspns) homemade low GI vinaigrette dressing (see page 127)

Cook the wholewheat pasta according to the instructions on the packet. Drain and toss in the vinaigrette dressing. Drain the tuna and flake. Add the tuna to the pasta and chill.

Serve on a bed of lettuce with a few radishes as a garnish.

Veal in Breadcrumbs

Serves 2

- 2 egg whites
- 2 escalopes of veal
- 60 g (2 oz) wholegrain or sourdough breadcrumbs
- 60 g (2 oz) rapeseed or corn oil
- ½ lemon (to garnish)

Beat the egg white and dip the veal in it.. Then dip the veal in the breadcrumbs, pressing the breadcrumbs firmly to the meat. Leave to set in a fridge for about an hour. Heat the oil in a non-stick frying pan and fry the veal for about 5 minutes on each side. Garnish with lemon.

Apple and Lemon Compote

Serves 4

- 455 g (1 lb) cooking apples
- 30 ml (2 tbspns) lemon juice

- ❑ 2 cloves
- ❑ 285 ml (½ pint) water
- ❑ liquid sweetener to taste

Peel and core the apples and place in a pan with the lemon juice, water and cloves. Cook gently until the fruit is soft, and then remove the cloves.

Serve hot or cold.

Tuna Salad

Serves 4

- ❑ 1 x 7 oz tin tuna in brine
- ❑ 1 lettuce
- ❑ 2 tomatoes
- ❑ ½ cucumber
- ❑ 4 spring onions

Arrange a couple of lettuce leaves on each plate. Slice the tomatoes and cucumber and arrange these on top of the lettuce. Flake the tuna fish and divide it between each plate. Chop the spring onions and sprinkle over the top.

Diet feature:

Tuna in brine has much less fat compared with tuna in oil.

Mushroom Marinade

Serves 4

- ❑ 225 g (8 oz) button mushrooms
- ❑ 1 clove garlic, crushed
- ❑ 5 g (1 tspn) chopped parsley
- ❑ 15 ml (1 tbspn) unsweetened tomato purée
- ❑ 85 ml (3 oz) white wine vinegar
- ❑ 5 ml (1 tspn) Worcestershire sauce
- ❑ 2.5 g (½ tspn) mustard powder
- ❑ 2.5 ml (½ tspn) liquid sweetener
- ❑ 55 ml (2 oz) water

- pinch of salt
- freshly ground black pepper

Slice the mushrooms and place them in a bowl. Mix all the marinade ingredients together and pour over the mushrooms. Season to taste. Cover with clear food wrap and leave in the fridge to marinade overnight. Give the mushrooms a good stir around two or three times while marinading. Next day drain off the liquid, put the mushrooms into a serving dish and sprinkle with parsley.

This salad can be served either as a starter or as a salad accompaniment.

Chicken with Basmati Rice

Serves 4

- 455 g (1 lb) cooked chicken breasts
- 1 green pepper
- 4 sticks celery
- 1 medium onion
- 115 g (4 oz) mushrooms (sliced)
- 170 g (6 oz) basmati rice
- 1 clove garlic (crushed)
- rapeseed or corn oil for cooking
- pinch of salt
- freshly ground black pepper

Dice the chicken and put one side. Cook the rice as directed on the packet. Meanwhile slice the vegetables into even-sized pieces. Heat the rapeseed or corn oil in a frying pan and fry the onion and garlic for three minutes. Add the green pepper and celery and cook for a further five minutes. Add the chicken, mushrooms, salt and pepper. Cover and cook gently for another five minutes. When the rice is cooked mix the rice and chicken and vegetable mixture together.

Serve with a salad.

Raspberry Sorbet

Serves 4

- 455 g (1 lb) raspberries
- 2 egg whites
- granulated or liquid sweetener

Make a purée out of the raspberries, saving about 10, and then sieve to remove the seeds. Sweeten to taste. Beat the egg whites until stiff and then fold into the purée mixture. Pour into a freezing tray and freeze for about two hours. Turn the mixture into a bowl and mash until smooth. Return it to the freezer and freeze until solid.

Serve decorated with two or three raspberries on each portion.

Mushroom and Onion Bake

Serves 2

- 225 g (8 oz) mushrooms, chopped
- 1 medium onion, chopped
- 2 large eggs
- 275 ml (½ pint) skimmed milk or soya milk
- rapeseed or corn oil for cooking
- pinch of salt
- freshly ground black pepper

(Similar to quiche but without the pastry.)

Heat the oil in a saucepan, add the onion and soften for a few minutes. Add the mushrooms and cook for about 20 minutes, stirring occasionally. Arrange evenly in the bottom of a greased dish. Whisk the eggs and milk together, and season with salt and pepper. Pour the eggs over the mushrooms and bake in a pre-heated oven, gas mark 4, 350°F (180°C), for about 35 minutes, until the centre is set. (If you like you can add a few courgettes or tomatoes or any vegetable you have before you add the eggs.) Serve immediately.

Roast Lamb with Garlic

Serves 4

- 1360 g (3lb) leg of lamb
- 2 cloves garlic
- 5 g (1 tspn) rosemary
- 5 g (1 tspn) thyme
- 2 sweet potatoes (cut into chunks) or 8-12 new potatoes
- 3 onions
- pinch of salt
- freshly milled black pepper
- 285 ml (½ pint) meat stock

Cut the garlic into small slivers and, using a sharp knife, make slits at 5 cm (2-inch) intervals all over the leg and insert the garlic into the slits. Rub the herbs all over the leg and place it in a roasting tin in a pre-heated oven, gas mark 8, 450°F (230°C), for 30 minutes. Meanwhile peel and slice the onions and potatoes, place in a large bowl, and season with salt and pepper. Layer the potatoes and onions around the leg in the tin, pour the hot stock over the vegetables, and return the tin to the oven for a further 1½ hours, reducing the temperature if the potatoes seem to be browning too quickly.

Serve with fresh mint sauce.

This is a delicious way of serving a joint without gravy.

Chocolate Soufflé

Serves 4

- 30 g (2 tbspns) cocoa powder
- 30 g (2 tbspns) cornflour
- 10 ml (2 tspns) liquid sweetener
- 430 ml (¾ pint) skimmed milk
- 55 ml (4 extra tbspns) skimmed milk
- 3 egg whites
- 5 ml (1 tspn) vanilla essence

Heat the 430 ml (3/4 pint) of skimmed milk. Carefully mix the cornflour, cocoa powder and sweetener with the 55 ml (4 tablespoons) of cold skimmed milk to form a smooth paste. Gently add to the hot milk and cook, stirring all the time, until the mixture thickens. Remove from the heat and allow to cool. Whip the egg whites with the vanilla essence until stiff and fold into the cold chocolate mixture. Spoon the mixture into a serving dish.

Serve chilled and decorated with a little grated chocolate.

Lamb Kebabs

Serves 4

- ❑ 455 g (1lb) leg of lamb
- ❑ 1 onion
- ❑ 1 green pepper
- ❑ 4 small tomatoes
- ❑ 2 cloves garlic, crushed
- ❑ 5 g (1 tspn) dried mixed herbs
- ❑ juice of 2 lemons
- ❑ pinch of salt
- ❑ freshly ground black pepper

Cut all the visible fat off the lamb and cut the meat into large cubes. Place the meat in a bowl, add the garlic and herbs, and season with salt and pepper. Pour the lemon juice over the mixture. Peel the onion and cut into quarters. Cut the green pepper into even-sized pieces. Add the onion and pepper to the meat mixture and stir well. Cover with cling film and leave for a few hours to marinade. Take a skewer and thread the meat on to it, alternating with a piece of onion and a piece of pepper, until the skewer is nearly full. Do the same with three more skewers and put a tomato on to the end of each skewer. Grill each skewer under a pre-heated grill, turning frequently, for 15 to 20 minutes, until the meat is well done.

These kebabs are also delicious cooked on a barbecue when they can be served with new potatoes or basmati rice.

Chicken Casserole

Serves 4

- ❑ 4 chicken breasts
- ❑ 455 g (1lb) carrots
- ❑ 455 g (1 lb) leeks.
- ❑ 4-6 small new potatoes
- ❑ 1 medium onion
- ❑ 2 cloves garlic (crushed)
- ❑ 2 sticks celery
- ❑ 570 ml (1 pint) chicken stock
- ❑ 15 ml (1 tbspn) rapeseed or corn oil

Prepare the vegetables by peeling and slicing into even sized pieces. Heat the oil in a large heavy casserole. Fry the chicken pieces until they are golden. Remove the chicken and place on a warm plate. Gently fry all the vegetables in the casserole for five minutes and add the garlic. Return the chicken to the casserole, placing them on top of the softened vegetables. Pour the chicken stock over the chicken and cook in the oven, gas mark 2, 300°F (150°C), for 2½ hours. This dish needs no accompanying vegetables.

Carrot and Onion Soup

Serves 4

- ❑ 2 onions
- ❑ 455 g (1lb) carrots
- ❑ 1 clove garlic
- ❑ 850 ml (1½ pints) beef stock
- ❑ 15 ml (1 tbspn) olive oil
- ❑ 30 ml (2 tbspns) low fat natural yoghurt
- ❑ pinch of salt
- ❑ freshly ground black pepper

Peel and thinly slice the carrots. Skin and chop the onion. Skin and crush the garlic. Melt the oil in a large saucepan. Fry the vegetables and garlic for 5 minutes. Add the beef stock, salt and pepper. Bring to the boil and simmer for

20 minutes. Liquidise the soup. Reheat in a saucepan. Stir in yoghurt before serving.

Red Cabbage Crunchy Salad

Serves 4

- ❑ 85 g (3 oz) red cabbage
- ❑ 3 sticks celery
- ❑ 1 apple
- ❑ ½ green pepper
- ❑ 30 ml (1 oz) low fat natural yoghurt
- ❑ 15 ml (1 tbspn) homemade low GI mayonnaise (see recipe, page 127)

Shred the cabbage, chop the celery and green pepper, core and slice the apple (and dip in lemon juice to prevent discoloration) and place the ingredients in a bowl. Add the yoghurt and vinaigrette and toss well.

Cod with Cucumber

Serves 4

- ❑ 4 x 170g (6 oz) cod steaks
- ❑ 170 g (6 oz) cucumber
- ❑ 1 lemon
- ❑ 55 g (2 oz) cottage cheese
- ❑ 140 g (5 oz) low-fat natural yoghurt
- ❑ pinch of salt
- ❑ freshly ground black pepper

Grate the lemon and then squeeze the juice from it. Place the fish in an ovenproof dish and add the lemon rind and juice. Cover and cook in a preheated oven, gas mark 4, 350°F (180°C), for 25 minutes. Drain off any excess liquid. Dice the cucumber and mix it with the cheese, yoghurt, salt and pepper. Heat the mixture and serve on top of the fish.

Serve garnished with sliced cucumber and parsley.

Orange and Rhubarb

Serves 4

- ❑ 455 g (1lb) rhubarb
- ❑ 2 oranges
- ❑ liquid or granulated sweetener

Cut the rhubarb into even-sized pieces about one inch long. Peel and slice the oranges. Layer the rhubarb and sliced oranges in casserole dish. Cover and bake in the oven, gas mark 3, 325°F (165°C), until the rhubarb is tender (about 30 minutes). Add the sweetener if required when cooked.

Serve hot or cold.

Vegetable Curry

Serves 4

- ❑ 450 g (1 lb) diced vegetables of your choice
- ❑ homemade curry sauce (see page 80)

If cauliflower or broccoli are required in addition, cut into florets and leave to one side.

Place the vegetables in an oven tray or casserole and cover with homemade curry sauce. Cook according to the vegetables you have used: only add cauliflower or broccoli for the final 10 minutes.

Serve with steamed or boiled basmati or wild rice.

Chicken Peppery Pasta

Serves 2

- ❑ 100 g chicken breast with skin and fat removed
- ❑ 1 dried apricot
- ❑ 50 g pasta of your choice
- ❑ 15 g (1tspn) Parmesan cheese
- ❑ olive oil for cooking
- ❑ pinch of parsley

- ❑ pinch of oregano
- ❑ pinch of crushed ground pepper
- ❑ small bowl of green salad

Slice and season the chicken to taste. Sauté in a non-stick frying pan, then add the pasta, pre-cooked *al dente.* Toss in further seasoning and add the Parmesan cheese and chopped apricot.

Serve with the green salad.

Plum and Pear Compote

Serves 4

- ❑ 225 g (8 oz) plums
- ❑ 225 g (8 oz) pears (peeled and sliced)
- ❑ 140 ml (¼ pint) water
- ❑ cinnamon
- ❑ liquid sweetener to taste

Halve the plums and remove the stones. Place the plums, pears and water in a pan. Cook gently until the fruit is soft and add the sweetener to taste.

Serve hot or cold with a sprinkling of cinnamon.

Lentil Soup

Serves 6

- ❑ 225 g (8 oz) lentils
- ❑ 1 onion
- ❑ 2 carrots
- ❑ 225 g (8 oz) tinned tomatoes
- ❑ rapeseed or corn for cooking
- ❑ 2 cloves garlic (crushed)
- ❑ 2 pints stock parsley

There is a bewildering array of lentils (there are literally dozens of varieties) on the market. My advice is to follow the cooking instructions on the packet of lentils that you buy.

Skin and chop the onion. Peel and chop the carrots. Heat the rapeseed or corn oil in a saucepan and fry the onion and carrots for 5 minutes. Add the remaining ingredients. Bring to the boil and simmer gently for about 1 hour (depending on the type of lentil).

This soup can be served as it is or else you can liquidise it if you prefer a smooth soup. Sprinkle with parsley and season to taste.

Incidentally, lentils are an excellent source of good protein. Although they are relatively deficient in sulphur-containing amino-acids they are rich in another essential amino-acid, lysine, in which many cereals are deficient. For this reason a combination of lentils and cereal provides a complete protein that compares well with animal protein. So it is a good idea to have a slice of wholegrain or sourdough bread with this soup.

Celery, Radish and Green Pepper Salad

Serves 4

- ❑ 4 sticks celery
- ❑ 12 radishes
- ❑ 1 green pepper
- ❑ 15 ml (1 tbspn) homemade low GI vinaigrette dressing (see recipe in this book) or lemon juice

Slice the celery into small, even pieces, and slice the radishes and green pepper. Mix together in a bowl and add vinaigrette or lemon juice.

Serve as a snack or as an accompaniment to snacks or main meals.

Grilled Sole with Grapes

Serves 4

- ❑ 4 x 170 g (6 oz) lemon soles
- ❑ 115 g (4 oz) green grapes
- ❑ 60 ml (4 tbspns) lemon juice
- ❑ 30 g (1 oz) rapeseed or corn oil
- ❑ chopped parsley
- ❑ freshly ground black pepper

Put a little of the oil on each sole and season with pepper. Grill for about 10 minutes, turning once. Meanwhile halve the grapes and remove the pips. When the fish is cooked serve with lemon juice and chopped parsley sprinkled over it and garnish with grapes.

Serve with mixed salad and new potatoes.

Apple and Blackberry Compote

Serves 4

- ❑ 225 g (8 oz) apples
- ❑ 225 g (8 oz) blackberries
- ❑ 140 ml (¼ pint) water
- ❑ liquid sweetener to taste

Peel and slice the apples and wash the blackberries. Put the fruit in a pan with the water, cook gently until the fruit is soft, and add the sweetener.

Serve hot or cold.

French Onion Soup

Serves 4

- ❑ 15 g (½ oz) rapeseed or corn oil
- ❑ 455 g (1lb) onions
- ❑ 2 cloves garlic, crushed
- ❑ 2.5 g (½ tspn) low-calorie granulated sweetener
- ❑ 850 ml (1½ pints) beef stock
- ❑ freshly ground black pepper

Heat the oil in a large saucepan. Slice the onions and add to the oil. Stir in the garlic, add the sweetener, and cook over a low heat for 15 minutes until the onions brown. Pour on the stock, bring to the boil, cover and simmer gently for 30 minutes. Season to taste and sprinkle with parsley.

Red Pepper and Beanshoot Salad

Serves 4

- ❑ 1 red pepper
- ❑ 225 g (8 oz) beanshoots
- ❑ 30 ml (2 tbspns) homemade low GI vinaigrette dressing (see recipe on page 127)

Finely slice the pepper and put it into a bowl with the beanshoots. Add the vinaigrette dressing and toss well.

Serve with a meat or a fish dish.

Chicken Curry

Serves 4

- ❑ 4 breasts of chicken with skin and fat removed, left whole or diced as required

Place in a saucepan or oven tray and cover with homemade curry sauce (see page 80). Cook gently until tender.

Serve with steamed or boiled basmati or wild rice.

Lemon Jelly with Banana

Serves 4

- ❑ 1 banana
- ❑ 1 packet of sugar-free lemon jelly
- ❑ juice of 1 lemon

Make the jelly as instructed on the packet. Stir in the lemon juice and allow to cool. Slice the banana thinly. Pour a layer of jelly, half an inch to an inch deep, into a mould and allow to set. Keep the rest of the jelly warm so it doesn't set. Arrange the banana slices over the set jelly and then carefully pour the remaining jelly mixture over the banana. Allow to set.

Unmould to serve.

Chilli Bean and Frankfurter Salad

Serves 4

- ❑ 1 x 420 g (15 oz) can red kidney beans, drained
- ❑ 1 red pepper
- ❑ 1 green pepper
- ❑ 1 onion
- ❑ 2 tomatoes
- ❑ 1 head chicory or lettuce
- ❑ 4 Frankfurters

Dressing:

- ❑ 30 ml (2 tbspns) homemade low GI vinaigrette dressing (see recipe on page 127)
- ❑ 2.5 ml (½ tspn) Tabasco sauce
- ❑ pinch chilli powder
- ❑ salt
- ❑ freshly ground black pepper

Peel and slice the onion, and slice the peppers and tomatoes. Drain and rinse the kidney beans. Cut the Frankfurters into bite-size pieces. Put all the ingredients into a large bowl. Mix together the ingredients of the dressing and pour over the bean mixture. Stir well and chill.

Serve on a bed of lettuce or chicory.

Haddock in Parsley Sauce

Serves 4

- ❑ 4 x 170 g (6 oz) haddock fillets
- ❑ 285 ml (10 oz) low-fat natural yoghurt
- ❑ 20 ml (4 tspns) lemon juice
- ❑ 60 g (4 tbspns) chopped parsley
- ❑ pinch of salt
- ❑ freshly ground black pepper

Poach the fish in a little water or grill for 10 to 15 minutes until tender. To make the sauce mix the yoghurt and lemon juice together and carefully heat but do not allow to boil. Season the mixture and add the chopped parsley.

Serve the fish with the sauce spooned over it.

Hot Fruit Compote

Serves 4

- 2 large oranges
- 2 large pears
- 1 apple
- 225 g (8 oz) fresh or frozen raspberries
- 140 ml (¼ pint) water
- liquid sweetener to taste
- cinnamon

Peel the oranges and divide into segments. Peel the pears and apple and cut into slices. Place the fruit in a saucepan with the water and cook gently for about 10 minutes, then add the sweetener and a sprinkling of cinnamon.

Serve hot with low-fat natural yoghurt or custard made with skimmed milk or soya milk and artificial sweetener.

Celery Soup

Serves 2

- 1 head of celery
- 30 ml (2 tbspns) low fat natural yoghurt
- 15 ml (1 tbspn) olive oil
- 2 beef or chicken stock cubes
- 570 ml (1 pint) water

Wash the celery and chop into small pieces. Lightly fry the celery for 5 minutes in the oil in a saucepan. Dissolve the stock cubes in hot water. Pour over the celery and cook until tender (about 30 minutes). Liquidise, return to pan, and stir in the yoghurt. Season if necessary.

Cucumber Jelly

Serves 6

- ❑ 1 cucumber
- ❑ 2 lemons
- ❑ 5 g (1 tspn) chopped mint
- ❑ 5 g (1 tspn) chopped thyme
- ❑ 285 g (10 oz) low fat natural yoghurt
- ❑ 15 g (½ oz) powdered gelatine
- ❑ pinch of salt
- ❑ freshly ground black pepper

Cut 2.5 cm (one inch) off the end of the cucumber, and thinly slice and arrange the slices in the bottom of a glass bowl. Peel the rest of the cucumber and dice. Grate the rind from the lemons and extract the juice. Dissolve the gelatine in 140 ml (¼ pint) cold water in a basin standing over a pan of simmering water. Stir in the lemon juice and rind, pour a thin layer of the lemon jelly into the glass bowl, and allow to set. Keeping the rest of the lemon mixture over the hot water stir it from time to time so that it does not set. When the bottom layer of the jelly is set whisk the yoghurt into the mixture in the basin, stir in the cucumber, mint and thyme, and season. Pour the mixture into the glass bowl and allow to set.

To serve dip the bowl in hot water and turn the jelly on to a plate. If you like, serve with lettuce.

Roast Beef and Wholemeal Yorkshire Pudding

Roasted meats, without any added fats, so beloved in many cookery books, are easy to cook and are an excellent way of preparing meat because some of the fat is lost during the cooking. Roast beef, served with horseradish sauce and low GI wholemeal Yorkshire Pudding (see recipe below), is delicious.

Wholemeal Yorkshire Pudding

Serves 6

- ❑ 115 g (4 oz) wholemeal flour
- ❑ 1 egg
- ❑ 285 ml (½ pint) skimmed milk or soya milk
- ❑ 15 g (½ oz) rapeseed or corn oil
- ❑ pinch of salt

Make the batter either by sieving the flour and salt into a mixing bowl, adding the milk and egg and mixing to a smooth batter or by mixing the same ingredients in a blender or food mixer. Heat the oil in a Yorkshire pudding tin in a pre-heated oven, gas mark 7, 425°F (220°C), until the fat is hot. Pour in the batter and cook for about 30 minutes.

Crêpes Suzette

Serves 4 to 6, depending on greed

- ❑ 4 oz (110 g) part plain and part wholemeal flour
- ❑ 1 oz (30 ml) olive oil
- ❑ 3 oz (85 g) polyunsaturated margarine
- ❑ finely grated rind of 2 medium-sized oranges
- ❑ 6 tbsps granulated artificial sweetener
- ❑ 2 tbsps Cointreau or Grand Marnier
- ❑ 1 egg
- ❑ 1 tbsp cooking brandy
- ❑ ½ pint skimmed milk

Make the batter either by sieving the flour and half the sweetener into a mixing bowl and adding the milk and egg and mixing to a smooth batter or by mixing the same ingredients in a blender or food mixer. Using a non-stick frying pan cook wafer-thin pancakes, using a minute amount of oil to grease the pan. If you use a 7-inch pan you should get about 12 pancakes. Stack them using greaseproof paper to prevent them sticking to each other. Now make the Suzette sauce by creaming together the margarine, the rest of the sweetener, orange rind and orange liqueur. Spread the sauce evenly over each pancake and roll each pancake up. Place the pancakes side by side in a flameproof dish and place in a pre-heated oven, gas mark 7, 220°C, 425°F, for 10 minutes. Bring to the table, pour the brandy from a well-heated ladle over the pancakes, and ignite (having first switched off the room lights). Spoon the liqueur and sauce over the pancakes, and serve.

Low GI Diet features:

Although this recipe is a bit of a diet breaker it has some good low GI diet features:

- Using skimmed milk instead of whole milk
- Using artificial sweetener instead of sugar
- Using part wholemeal flour instead of all plain flour

It is important to indulge in 'forbidden' foods occasionally, but at the same time it makes sense to do so in the healthiest way possible. This dish is one of my own favourites and is always a great hit at dinner parties.

Home-Made Low GI Mayonnaise

- ❑ 285 ml (½ pint) skimmed milk or soya milk
- ❑ 15 g (½ oz) cornflour
- ❑ 7.5g (1½ tspn) dry mustard
- ❑ 5 g (1 tspn) paprika
- ❑ 12 drops liquid sweetener
- ❑ pinch of salt
- ❑ 100 ml (6 tbspns) extra virgin olive oil
- ❑ 100 ml (6 tbspns) vinegar or lemon juice

Mix the milk and cornflour together in a saucepan to make a paste, and cook until thickened. Place the paste in a bowl, add the mustard, paprika, sweetener and salt, and beat the ingredients until smooth. Gradually add the oil and vinegar (or lemon juice), beating all the time, until the mixture is blended.

Home-Made Low GI Vinaigrette Dressing

- ❑ 40 ml (3 tbspns) wine vinegar
- ❑ 15 ml (1 tbspn) extra virgin olive oil

- ❑ 5 ml (1 tspn) Worcestershire sauce
- ❑ 5 g dry mustard
- ❑ 2 drops liquid sweetener

Put the ingredients into a screw-top jar and shake well.

Chapter 19

Some Common Carbohydrate Foods and their GI Values

This is the part you will find yourself referring to time and again. So it's important to bear several points in mind.

First, in the LOW GI column, foods in CAPITALS have especially low GI values.

Second, some foods, although with low GI values, have amounts of fat which exceed the recommended guidelines.

Third, only carbohydrates have GI values. So meat, for example, which is made of protein and fat but contains no carbohydrate, has no GI value.

Fourth – and this is the most important – the GI value of a food is not the be all and end all. Watermelon, for example, has a high GI. But combine it with several other fruits with low GI values and the overall GI value of such a fruit salad is low. The overall value of a combination of foods is called its glycaemic load or GL.

Another way to reduce the overall glycaemic load of a meal is to combine carbohydrates with non-carbohydrates. For example, spaghetti on its own or with a tomato-based sauce has a higher glycaemic load than spaghetti Bolognese. This is because the meat has no GI. In fact, it is very important to try to combine protein with carbohydrate as much as you can. Protein is slowly digested which both reduces the glycaemic load of the meal and also satisfies hunger more easily. This is one reason why high protein diets help weight loss – you actually feel less hungry.

Finally remember that the GI values in the next few pages are approximate. The GI value of a fruit, for example, will vary with its ripeness. The GI value of pasta will depend on how well cooked it is. So GI is not an exact science, but it is a good guide. If you use it sensibly it will help you to both control your weight and to eat a diet that is kind to your heart and your body's metabolism.

GI VALUES OF SOME COMMON CARBOHYDRATE FOODS

	LOW GI	MEDIUM GI	HIGH GI
BISCUITS	Oatmeal	Shortbread	Morning coffee
BREADS	Pumpernickel	Croissant (contains significant fat)	Bagel
	Sourdough	Crumpet	Baguette
	100% stoneground whole wheat	Pita bread, whole wheat	Dark rye
		Rye	Gluten-free
		Whole wheat, not stoneground	Melba toast
			White
			Wholemeal bread
CEREALS	All-Bran	Mini Wheats	Bran Flakes
	Muesli, toasted	Muesli, natural	Coco Pops
	Porridge (not instant)	Nutri-grain	Corn flakes
	Special K	Porridge, instant	Weetabix
			Rice Krispies
			Shredded Wheat
			Sultana Bran
CONFEC-TIONERY	Chocolate (contains significant fat)	Mars bar (contains significant fat)	Jelly beans
		Muesli bar (contains significant fat)	
CONVEN-IENCE FOODS	Fish fingers		
	Sausages (contain significant fat)		

	LOW GI	**MEDIUM GI**	**HIGH GI**
CRACKERS		Ryvita	Crispbread
			Rice cakes
			Water crackers
DAIRY	Custard	Condensed milk, sweetened	
	Ice cream, low fat	Ice cream, full fat	
	Milk, whole, semi-skimmed or skimmed		
	Soy milk		
	Yoghurt, with sugar, with or without fruit		
	Yoghurt, with sweetener, with or without fruit		

	LOW GI	MEDIUM GI	HIGH GI
FRUIT	Apple	Apricots, fresh or canned	Dates, dried
	Apricots (Dried)	Apricot jam	Lychee
	Cherries	Banana	Watermelon
	Fruit cocktail	Kiwi fruit	
	Grapefruit	Melon	
	Grapes	Mango	
	Orange	Papaya	
	Orange marmalade	Peach, canned	
	Peach, fresh	Pineapple	
	Pear, fresh or canned	Raisins	
	Plum	Sultanas	
	Prunes		
	Strawberries		
	Strawberry jam		
FRUIT JUICES	Apple juice		
	Grapefruit juice		
	Orange juice		
	Pineapple juice, unsweetened		
LEGUMES	Baked beans		Broad beans
	Butter beans		
	Chickpeas		
	Haricot beans		
	Kidney Beans		
	Lentils		
	Soya Beans		

	LOW GI	**MEDIUM GI**	**HIGH GI**
RICE	Converted, Uncle Ben's	Basmati, boiled	Instant
	Parboiled	Brown	Rice cakes
		Long grain, white	Short grain, white
			Sticky
SNACKS	Peanuts (contain significant fat)	Potato crisps (contain significant fat)	Popcorn
SUGARS	Fructose	Honey	Glucose
		Sucrose (table sugar)	
VEG	Carrots	Beetroot	Parsnip
	Peas	Small new potatoes	Potatoes
	Sweet corn		Pumpkin
	Sweet potato		Swede

Appendix

Grapefruit Interactions

Grapefruit can interact with some prescription medications either to increase the effect of those medications or to produce side-effects. Something in grapefruit, perhaps a bioflavonoid, inhibits an enzyme, CYP 3A4, in the wall of the intestine, and this enzyme is important for the breakdown of hundreds of medications. When its effectiveness is compromised, blood levels of these drugs can rise and cause undesirable side-effects. This happens only with drugs taken by mouth – not those given by injection or via skin patch, and the effect may last for as long as two days. If you are on any of these drugs you should discuss this with your doctor who will help you to monitor any possible interactions.

Drugs which may interact with grapefruit in some people:

- Some calcium channel blockers eg Felodipine (Plendil), Nicardipine (Cardene), Nifedipine (Adalat), Verapamil.
- Some heart drugs eg Amiodarone (Cordarone), Quinidine.
- Some statins eg Atorvastatin (Lipitor), Simvastatin (Zocor) but not Pravastatin (Pravachol) and fluvastatin (Lescol).
- The blood pressure drug, losartan (Cozaar).
- Some sleeping pills and anti-anxiety drugs eg Buspirone, (Buspar), Diazepam (Valium), Triazolam (Halcion).
- Some transplant drugs eg Cyclosporine, Tacrolimus and Sirolimus.
- Some antidepressants eg nefazodone (Serzone) and trazodone (Desyrel).
- The antipsychotic, clomipramine (Anafranil).
- The cortosone-like drug, methylprednisolone.
- The impotence (erectile dysfunction) drug, sildenafil (Viagra).
- The asthma drug, montelukast (Singulair).
- The Alzheimer's drug, donepezil (Aricept).

- The breast cancer drug, tamoxifen (Nolvadex).
- The prostate drug, tamsulosin (Flomax).
- The antihistamines loratadine (Claritin) and fexofenadine (Allegra).
- Some oestrogens.
- Some birth control pills.
- The HIV/AIDS drugs, Ritonavir (Norvir), Saquinavir (Fortovase, Invirase).
- The epilepsy drug, Carbamazepine (Tegretol).

THE DOCTOR'S DIET RECIPE BOOK

Recipes Containing Fructose

Please note that fructose can be obtained from many good health food shops.

Cabbage Soup

Serves 4 - 6

Ingredients

- 1 large savoy cabbage
- 200g smoked bacon
- 300g cured ham - thickly sliced
- 200g streaky bacon
- 4 small celeriac - diced
- 2 onions
- freshly ground pepper

Fill a large, heavy saucepan with 3 litres of water. Put into it the ham, smoked bacon and streaky bacon. Bring to the boil. Skim.

Remove any tired leaves from the cabbage. Remove the stem and cut the cabbage into four. Add to the stockpot, together with the diced celeriac and the peeled onions. Season with pepper. Reduce the heat, cover and allow to cook for a good 2 hours. Take out the meat and halve the vegetables, which will make up the main dish later. Put the remainder (liquid and vegetables) into the blender to make the soup. Serve very hot.

Cream of Radish Soup

Serves 4

Ingredients

- 2 bunches radishes with leaves
- 2 leeks
- 100ml low-fat crème fraîche
- 1 litre chicken stock
- salt, pepper
- 2 tbsp olive oil

Wash the radishes, complete with their leaves, and the leeks. Chop both finely and fry gently in the olive oil.

Bring the stock up to the boil and add to the vegetables. Cook on a high heat for 5 minutes. Blend to a purée and sieve.

Season with salt and pepper. Reheat the soup before serving and add the crème fraîche at the last minute.

Chilled Cucumber Soup

Serves 4

Ingredients

- 2 cucumbers
- 4–6 tbsp single cream
- ½ clove garlic
- 2 shallots
- 1 tbsp tarragon vinegar
- a few sprigs dill
- salt, pepper

Peel the cucumbers and cut them lengthways. Remove the seeds, cover with rough salt to draw out the liquid and put to one side.

Peel the garlic and shallots. Dry the cucumber with absorbent kitchen paper and blend with the garlic, shallots, vinegar and cream, to make a very smooth soup.

Season with salt and pepper and place in the refrigerator for one hour. Serve garnished with a few sprigs of dill.

Crab, Fish and Avocado Loaf

Serves 6

Ingredients

- 400g frozen fish sticks ('crab sticks', 'ocean sticks')
- 2 avocados
- 4 hard-boiled eggs
- 4 tbsp thick low-fat crème fraîche
- 4 tbsp chopped chervil
- 1 tin crab pieces
- 2 leaves (or 2 tsp powdered) gelatine
- juice of 1 lemon
- 1 tsp olive oil
- salt, pepper

Thaw the fish sticks in the refrigerator. Peel the avocados and remove the stones. Blend the flesh of the avocados with 2 tbsp of the crème fraîche. Season with the lemon juice, salt, pepper and chervil. Oil a loaf tin and line the bottom and sides with fish sticks. Reserve some to place on the top of the loaf. Chop the remainder of the fish sticks and the hard-boiled eggs.

Soften the gelatine leaves in cold water and drain. Heat the rest of the crème fraîche and dissolve the gelatine in it. Mix the chopped fish sticks and chopped egg together and combine with half the warm crème fraîche. Leave to cool until lukewarm. Drain the crab and add it to the remainder of the warm crème fraîche. Stir and leave to cool until lukewarm. Into the loaf tin pour a layer of the fish sticks mixture, followed by a layer of avocado mixture, a layer of crab mixture, a second layer of avocado mixture and, finally, a second layer of fish sticks mixture.

Place the remaining fish sticks on top and refrigerate for 12 hours.

Mushroom and Garlic Fromage Frais Mould

Serves 4

Ingredients

- 200g garlic
- 150g fromage frais
- 100g tinned button mushrooms
- 4 eggs
- 10g butter
- salt, pepper

Peel the garlic cloves and remove the central shoot. Steam or cook in a very little water for 20 minutes. Purée the garlic and mushrooms together in a blender.

Add the fromage frais and season with salt and pepper. Mix thoroughly until the purée is smooth and creamy. Then add the beaten eggs and a dash of salt.

Place the mixture in buttered ramekins and cook in a bain-marie for 20 minutes at 180°C, 350°F, Gas Mark 4. They are cooked when the tops feel firm to the touch.

Mousse of Parma Ham and Leeks

Serves 6

Ingredients

- 2kg leeks (white part only)
- 200g very thinly sliced Parma ham
- 1 bunch chives
- 30g butter
- 2 eggs
- 100g grated cheese
- salt, pepper
- 100ml low-fat crème fraîche

Wash the leeks, blanch for 10 minutes in boiling salted water and drain. Blend the Parma ham and add the eggs, lightly beaten, the cream and the grated cheese. Season with the salt, pepper and chopped chives.

Pour a layer of the mixture into a loaf tin and follow this with a layer of leeks. Continue in this way until the tin is filled. Place in the oven at 220°C, 425°F, Gas Mark 7 for 30 minutes. Serve in slices, hot or cold.

Suggestion: The discarded green parts of the leeks can be used in a vegetable soup.

Tomatoes Stuffed with Tuna

Serves 6

Ingredients

- 6 medium tomatoes
- 200g tuna in brine
- 500g fresh peas
- 200ml sunflower oil
- 1 tbsp olive oil
- 1 tsp Dijon mustard
- 2 garlic cloves
- 1 egg yolk
- 1 tbsp chopped parsley
- salt, pepper

Slice off the round end of the tomatoes, scoop out the inside with a small spoon (keep the flesh), and turn them upside down to drain.

Shell the peas and cook in boiling salted water for 2 minutes. Drain and allow to cool.

Make a mayonnaise, as follows:

Crush 3 cloves of garlic and combine with the egg yolk and mustard. Whisk in, a very little at a time, the 200ml sunflower oil, and then the tbspful of olive oil. Season with salt and pepper.

Drain and flake the tuna. Combine with the mayonnaise, peas and drained tomato flesh. Fill the tomatoes with the mixture, sprinkle with chopped parsley and replace the lids. Serve chilled.

French Vinaigrette

Prepared in a bottle or cruet

Ingredients

- 1 tbsp strong mustard
- 150ml wine vinegar
- 200ml sunflower oil
- 200ml olive oil
- 1 tsp sea salt
- 3 grindings of pepper
- 1 clove garlic, crushed
- 1 tsp Herbes de Provence
- 3 pinches mild paprika
- 1 small pinch cayenne
- 1 pinch curry powder

Dissolve all the solid ingredients in the vinegar. Add the oils and shake well.

Gourmand Salad

Serves 4

Ingredients

- 400g very fine French beans
- 8 scallops
- 200g foie gras
- 1 bunch parsley
- balsamic vinaigrette with olive oil
- sea salt, freshly ground pepper

If you cannot use fresh foie gras, then use the tinned version. Cut into 8 thin slices and arrange on a plate. Cover with plastic film and place in the fridge for at least an hour.

Cook the French beans so they remain slightly firm. Prepare the vinaigrette: dissolve the salt in the balsamic vinegar and add the pepper and olive oil. Mix well.

Poach the scallops for 5 minutes in water with the sea salt and pepper. Drain and reserve.

Just before serving, using a very sharp knife slice the scallops very thinly. Arrange the French beans edged with the sliced scallops on each plate, and then add the 2 slices of foie gras. Decorate with parsley and lace with the vinaigrette.

Celeriac and Avocado Remoulade

Serves 4

Ingredients

- 1 large celeriac weighing about 600g
- 1 ripe avocado
- 200g yoghurt
- 1 dozen black olives, stoned
- 1 lemon
- 1 tbsp strong mustard
- 3 tbsp olive oil
- 2 cloves garlic
- 1 tbsp powdered wheat germ
- 1 tbsp chopped parsley
- salt, freshly ground pepper, ground coriander

Peel the celeriac, cut into manageable lumps and grate. Sprinkle lemon juice over the top to prevent it oxidising and going brown.

Crush the garlic. Stone the avocado and scoop out the flesh.

To make the sauce: Put the avocado, yoghurt, mustard, wheat germ, olive oil, garlic and black olives into a food processor. Season with salt, pepper and a few pinches of coriander and blend for a few seconds to obtain a sauce with the consistency of a mayonnaise.

Mix the celeriac with the sauce.

Arrange in a serving dish or on individual plates, and decorate with chopped parsley.

Creamy Cucumber Salad

Serves 3 to 4

Ingredients

- 4 fresh pickling cucumbers, peeled and sliced
- 50ml plain yoghurt
- 50ml sour cream
- 15ml freshly squeezed lime juice
- 1 small clove garlic, peeled and crushed
- 15ml finely chopped fresh chives
- 15ml finely chopped cilantro
- ¼ tsp celery salt
- freshly ground black pepper to taste,

In a bowl, combine all ingredients. Refrigerate 1 hour, and serve.

Pork Chops with Cream of Mustard Sauce

Serves 4

Ingredients

- 4 large pork chops (or 8 small chops)
- 80g crème fraîche
- 3 tbsp strong French mustard
- 1 tbsp capers (preferably salted)
- 1 tbsp goose fat

In a bowl, mix the crème fraîche, mustard and rinsed capers. Over a medium to high heat, melt the goose fat in a large frying pan and brown the chops for 7 to 8 minutes on each side. Season with salt and pepper.

Pour the sauce over the chops. Cover the pan and allow to simmer for about 10 minutes.

Serve on warm plates.

Marinated Pork Chops

Serves 4

Ingredients

- olive oil
- 1 medium onion, finely chopped
- 6 medium very ripe tomatoes, peeled and coarsely chopped
- 1 large clove garlic, peeled and crushed
- 45ml pesto sauce
- 30ml freshly squeezed lime juice 1 tsp
- 1 tsp dried oregano
- 1 tsp dried tarragon
- 1 tsp celery salt
- ½ tsp coriander powder
- salt and pepper to taste
- 8 pork chops, grilled

Heat 2 tbsp olive oil in a large saucepan; add onions and cook over low heat for 3 minutes.

Add tomatoes together with 2 more tbsp olive oil and the rest of the ingredients (except pork chops). Mix the sauce thoroughly, partially cover and simmer 1 to 1½ hours, stirring occasionally. Refrigerate 10 to 12 hours.

Spoon sauce onto grilled pork chops before serving.

Note: To peel tomatoes, plunge into boiling water 30 seconds and remove; skin will peel off easily.

Pork Ragout with Cockles

Serves 4

Ingredients

- 800g shoulder or hand of pork
- 1 litre cockles
- 6 tbsp olive oil
- 4 cloves garlic
- juice of 1 lemon
- 1 tbsp chopped parsley
- salt, pepper

For the marinade

- 180 ml dry white wine
- 1 bay leaf
- 1 garlic clove
- 1 onion spiked with 1 clove
- 1 bouquet garni

Make a marinade with the white wine, the bay leaf, onion, salt, pepper and bouquet garni.

Cut the meat up, pour the marinade over it and leave it to marinate for a day. Wash the cockles very thoroughly, drain, open them up over a high heat and remove the shells.

Remove the meat from the marinade and dry on absorbent kitchen paper. In a flameproof casserole, brown the meat in olive oil on a high heat. Filter the marinade and remove the onion. Dry the onion on kitchen paper and slice, removing the clove. Add the onion and crushed garlic to the casserole to cook. Add the filtered marinade, cover and cook on low heat for 1½ hours.

Check the casserole from time to time, adding a little water as necessary and turning the meat over. Five minutes before the end of the cooking time, put the sauce through the blender and then add the cockles to it.

Add the lemon juice and chopped parsley to the sauce before serving.

Green Peppers Stuffed with Veal

Serves 4

Ingredients

- 8 medium green peppers
- 45ml olive oil
- 10 green onions, thinly sliced
- 500ml thinly sliced mushrooms
- 250ml thinly sliced celery
- 450g lean ground veal
- 2 cloves garlic, peeled and crushed
- 1 tsp dried Herbes de Provence
- 4 medium-size ripe tomatoes, diced
- 1 tsp undiluted vegetable stock
- 75ml hot water
- salt and pepper
- 175ml cooked green lentils
- 125ml freshly grated Parmesan cheese
- 250ml part-skim grated mozzarella cheese

Cut top off peppers, core and seed, and rinse well. Soak in hot water 4 minutes. Drain on paper towels and set aside.

Preheat oven to 190°C, 375°F, Gas Mark 5.

In a large skillet, heat olive oil and cook onions, mushrooms and celery over low heat 3 minutes. Add garlic and veal, and cook over medium heat until meat has browned.

Add tomatoes and stock thinned with the hot water. Season with salt and pepper; stir, and simmer about 8 minutes.

Add cooked lentils to the mixture and stir well. Fill each pepper halfway with the mixture and sprinkle with Parmesan. Fill peppers with remaining mixture and top with mozzarella.

Place filled peppers in a baking dish, and bake about 15 minutes or until cheese is golden.

Roast Veal with Olives

Serves 4/5

Ingredients

- joint of veal weighing about 1.2kg
- 100g streaky bacon - diced
- 200g black olives - stoned
- 200g green olives - stoned
- 150ml white wine
- salt, freshly ground pepper, thyme

In a casserole fry the diced streaky bacon over a gently heat. Add the veal and brown lightly all over. Season with salt, pepper and sprinkle with a few pinches of thyme. Cover and cook over a very gently heat.

Combine 1 tbsp of olive oil with 75g green olives and 75g black olives in a blender and reduce to a purée. Pour into the casserole and stir in the wine. Leave to cook over a gentle heat for 1 hour, turning the meat from time to time.

Add the rest of the olives and allow to cook for a further 20 to 30 minutes, always over a low heat.

Take the roast out of the casserole. Slice and arrange on a warm dish and garnish with the olives.

Pour off the juices and set aside. Deglaze the residue on the bottome of the casserole with a little boiling water. Add the juices and stir.

Pour into a sauceboat and serve.

Veal Brochettes

Serves 4

Ingredients

- 675g veal loin, bones and fat removed
- 16 small onions, peeled
- 1 medium courgette, sliced into 1 cm pieces
- 16 cherry tomatoes

Marinade

- 50ml olive oil
- 1 tbsp tamari sauce
- 2 tbsp grated fresh ginger
- 2 tsp curry powder

Cut the veal into 2.5cm cubes.In a large bowl, mix marinade ingredients, reserving a quarter for basting. Add veal and mix to coat well. Refrigerate about 3 hours. Boil onions in lightly salted water until tender.

Preheat broiler. Thread marinated veal onto metal skewers, alternating with the vegetables. Baste onions, courgette and tomatoes with rest of marinade. Place skewers in a shallow pan and broil about 15 minutes, turning over and basting halfway through cooking.

Fillet Steak with Mushrooms

Serves 4

Ingredients

- 4 thick fillet steaks (250g each)
- 4 shallots
- 2 onions
- 500g fresh button mushrooms
- 1 small sprig thyme
- 4 sprigs parsley
- 4 tbsp olive oil
- salt, pepper

Chop the onions, shallots and parsley together. Trim, wash and slice the mushrooms and cook for 5 to 8 minutes in olive oil on a high heat.

Then season with salt and pepper. Add the chopped onion mixture late in cooking.

Grill the steaks for 2 to 3 minutes each side. Season with salt and pepper.

Serve accompanied by the mushrooms.

Minced Beef in a Cheese Soufflé

Serves 6

Ingredients

- 1 green pepper
- 2 onions
- 100g fresh mushrooms
- 3 medium tomatoes
- 500g minced beef
- 1 pinch oregano or thyme
- 2 tbsp chopped fine herbs
- salt, pepper, cayenne pepper
- olive oil

For the soufflé

- 3 eggs
- 60g grated cheddar
- 3 tbsp low-fat crème fraîche
- salt, cayenne pepper

Wash and chop the peppers into small pieces. Slice the onions thinly and fry with the peppers on a high heat in olive oil. Then add the mushrooms, washed and sliced.

Plunge the tomatoes into boiling water for 30 seconds, skin, remove the seeds and chop. Add to the pan, together with the minced meat, the fine herbs and the oregano. Season with salt, pepper and a dash of cayenne.

Cook on a high heat, without a lid so that the liquid evaporates, then lower the heat and continue to simmer for a few minutes more.

Melt the cheese in a bain-marie and add the crème fraîche. Allow to cool slightly. Add the egg yolks and season with salt, pepper and cayenne.

Beat the egg whites until they form stiff peaks and fold gently into the cheese mixture.

Spread the meat and vegetables in the bottom of a dish and pour the egg mixture over. Cook in a gentle oven (150 °C, 300 °F, Gas Mark 2) for 20 to 25 minutes.

Serve the soufflé as soon as it is cooked.

Roast Beef with Red Wine

Serves 4 to 6

Ingredients

- 900g roast beef, bone removed
- 500ml water
- 80ml olive oil
- 80ml tamari sauce
- 15ml strawberry vinegar
- 15ml cider vinegar
- 4 cloves garlic, peeled and crushed
- ½ tsp dried oregano
- ½ tsp dried parsley flakes
- ½ tsp dried thyme
- freshly ground black pepper to taste
- 12 Brussels sprouts
- 225g wax beans, cut in half
- 125ml red wine

Preheat oven to 180 °C, 350 °F, Gas Mark 4. In a casserole, place beef. Add water, olive oil, tamari, both vinegars, garlic and seasonings. Cover and bake 30 minutes. Add Brussels sprouts and wax beans, cover, and bake 30 minutes more. Remove and slice beef into 1 cm slices. Return to casserole, spreading slices around, pour wine over, and roast, uncovered, 30 to 45 minutes, or until vegetables are crisp-tender. If necessary, add a little water during the cooking to prevent from drying.

Provençal Beef Casserole

Serves 6

Ingredients

- 1kg beef (preferably chuck)
- 2 medium onions
- ½ clove garlic
- 4 tbsp olive oil
- 1kg ripe tomatoes
- ½ tsp thyme leaves
- ½ bay leaf
- 2 tbsp chopped parsley
- salt, pepper, nutmeg
- 50g black olives

Peel the onions and slice thinly, and fry in olive oil on high heat.

Plunge the tomatoes into boiling water for 30 seconds, skin and remove the seeds. Add to the onions, along with the thyme, bay leaf, garlic and chopped parsley.

Turn down the heat, cover and simmer. Add the meat, cut into 3 cm cubes and seasoned with salt, pepper and nutmeg. Pour on a little water if necessary.

Cook gently for 2 hours over very low heat. Serve decorated with black olives, added 10 minutes before the end of the cooking time.

Lamb Curry

Serves 6

Ingredients

- 1.5kg shoulder of lamb with fat removed
- 3 good-sized onions
- 3 good-sized aubergines
- 1 pepper
- 1 tbsp cumin seeds
- 1 tbsp mustard seeds
- 2½ tbsp curry powder
- olive oil
- salt

Cut the meat into 3cm pieces. Then, in a flameproof casserole, fry the chopped onions in olive oil over a low heat for 3 minutes.

Add the cumin and mustard seeds and stir for 2 minutes. Add the meat and brown, then salt lightly. Sprinkle on the curry powder, stirring it in.

Add 50ml of hot water, cover and leave to simmer for just over an hour.

Thirty-five minutes into the cooking time, add the aubergines (chopped and with the skin left on) and the diced pepper.

Adjust the seasoning as necessary at the end of cooking. Add a drizzle of olive oil a few minutes before serving.

English Leg of Lamb – French Style

Serves 5

Ingredients

- 1.5kg leg of lamb
- 2 bunches mint
- 1 tbsp fructose
- 1 glass cider vinegar
- goose fat
- salt, freshly ground pepper, cayenne

Grease the roasting tin with goose fat. Cover the bottom of the tin with mint leaves. Brush the leg liberally with goose fat. Season with salt, pepper and dust very lightly with cayenne all over.

Cook in the oven (190°C, 375°F, Gas Mark 5) for 1 hour 30 or 40 minutes, depending on how pink you prefer your lamb.

While the meat is cooking, chop finely two dozen leaves of mint. Boil the cider vinegar in a pan together with the chopped mint for 2 minutes. Turn off the heat and allow to cool for 3 minutes.

Add the fructose, stirring well to ensure that it dissolves completely. Liquidise. Then place in the refrigerator to chill. Remove the leg of lamb from the oven and carve in the tin, to ensure none of the juices are lost. Then arrange the meat on a hot serving dish.

Deglaze the cooking tin with a glass of boiling salted water and pour into a sauce boat. Serve the meat at the same time as the mint sauce and the deglazed cooking juices.

Sautéed Turkey

Serves 6

Ingredients

- 1.2kg turkey breast fillets
- 4 large onions
- 6 tomatoes
- 3 red peppers
- 2 tbsp sweet paprika
- 1 pinch cayenne pepper
- 4 tbsp olive oil or goose fat
- salt, pepper

Plunge the tomatoes into boiling water for 30 seconds, skin and remove the seeds. Fry the chopped onions in 2 tbsp olive oil. When they are golden, add the peppers, cut into strips, and the tomatoes.

Cook the mixture on low heat until it has turned into a purée. Season with salt, pepper, a pinch of cayenne and the paprika.

Slice the turkey fillets, not too thinly, into escalopes. Fry on a high heat in 2 tbsp olive oil or goose fat.

When they are just about cooked through but not too well done, turn down the heat and simmer for a few minutes more.

Serve right away with the vegetable purée.

Turkey with Apples

Serves 8

Ingredients

- 1 turkey weighing 3.5kg
- 600g sliced onions
- 1.5kg apples (Cox)
- 4 cloves garlic - chopped
- 6 leaves fresh sage
- goose fat
- olive oil
- 1 lemon
- salt, freshly ground pepper, cayenne
- 1 glass cider
- 200ml double cream

In a frying pan brown the onions in olive oil. Add the garlic towards the end. Peel and quarter the apples. Squeeze lemon over them to prevent them turning brown. Cook one third of the apples in the goose fat over a low heat. Chop the sage and add to the onions, garlic and apples to make a stuffing. Season with salt, pepper and cayenne. Stuff the turkey and sew up the opening. Coat the turkey with the goose fat. Season with salt, pepper and sprinkle lightly with cayenne.

Put in a roasting tin, adding a good glass of water and place in a fairly hot oven (190°C, 375°F, Gas Mark 5). Cook for 2 hours and 15 minutes, basting every 30 minutes. During the last half hour, pour off the cooking juices and add the rest of the peeled and quartered apples. Pour a quarter of the cooking juices carefully over the apples, reserving the rest to make the sauce. When the turkey is done, deglaze the roasting tin with the cider, stirring in the reserved juices together with the double cream.

Duck Breasts in Green Pepper Sauce

Serves 4

Ingredients

- 4 duck breasts
- 200g mushrooms
- 1 lemon
- 100ml red wine
- 1 onion
- 1 bay leaf
- 30 green peppercorns
- 1 tbsp olive or sunflower oil

Slice the onions and soften in 1 tbsp olive (or sunflower) oil. Add the red wine. Leave on a high heat until the liquid has almost completely evaporated.

Add 1 glass of water, the bay leaf and green pepper and cook for 15 minutes.

Trim and wash the mushrooms and cook whole in water with the lemon juice for 5 minutes. Blend to a purée, season with salt and add the butter. Strain the sauce through a sieve and return to a low heat to reduce. Add the mushroom purée.

Cook the duck breasts in a non-stick frying pan with no added fat or oil. Allow 4 minutes each side on a medium heat.

The duck breasts can be sliced into long, thin strips. Serve covered with the sauce.

Duck Breasts with Olives

Serves 4

Ingredients

- 500g green olives - stoned
- 4 duck breasts
- salt, freshly ground pepper, cayenne
- olive oil

Purée 200g olives in the blender with 1 tbsp of olive oil.

Remove three-quarters of the fat covering the duck. Use a third of the fat. Cut into cubes and melt slowly over a low heat. Discard the residue.

Add the olive purée. Season with salt and pepper, then add the rest of the olives and cook for 5 minutes.

For pink centres, fry the duck breasts in a non-stick pan for 6 minutes each side, starting with the fatty side. Vary the cooking time according to taste. Turn off the heat.

Cut the breasts into slices 1cm thick, coat with the olive purée and serve on warm plates.

Chicken Croquettes

Serves 2 to 3

Ingredients

- 450g ground chicken breast
- 1 large egg, beaten
- 50ml freshly grated Parmesan cheese
- 2 tbsp oat bran
- 1 large clove garlic, peeled and crushed
- 1 tsp dried Herbes de Provence
- 1 tsp nutmeg powder
- salt and freshly ground pepper to taste
- olive oil

In a bowl, combine ground chicken, egg, Parmesan, bran, garlic and seasonings. Shape into 8 croquettes.

Preheat oven to 220°C, 425°F, Gas Mark 7.

Place croquettes on a baking sheet lightly greased with olive oil. Bake 12 to 15 minutes, or until chicken is no longer pink when tested with a fork. Broil a few minutes to finish cooking when croquettes will be golden.

Chicken Breasts in a Creamy Garlic Sauce

Serves 4

Ingredients

- 4 boneless chicken breasts
- 2 heads garlic
- 300ml soya cream
- goose fat
- salt, freshly ground pepper, mild paprika
- cayenne
- 1 bunch parsley

Break up the heads of garlic, peel the cloves and cook in a steamer for 30 minutes. Place the chicken breasts in an ovenware dish and brush with goose fat. Season with salt and pepper and sprinkle lightly with cayenne. Put in the oven (190°C, 375°F, Gas Mark 5) for 20 to 25 minutes.

Liquidise the garlic cloves with the soya cream. Season with salt, pepper and add half a teaspoon of mild paprika.

Remove the chicken breasts from the oven and cut widthways in 1 to 2cm slices. Rearrange in the cooking dish. Coat with the garlic cream and leave in a lukewarm oven for 10 to 15 minutes. Sprinkle with chopped parsley and serve.

Indian-Style Chicken

Serves 4

Ingredients

- 125ml sour cream
- 2 tbsp freshly squeezed lime juice
- 15ml olive oil
- 2 tsp Dijon mustard
- 1½ tbsp grated fresh ginger
- 1 tsp coriander powder
- ½ tsp saffron powder
- ¼ tsp cumin powder
- salt and pepper to taste
- 4 chicken breasts, bones, fat and skin removed

In a shallow baking dish, combine all marinade ingredients. Add chicken, turning over to coat well. Marinate in refrigerator about 3 hours. Preheat oven to 180°C, 350°F, Gas Mark 4. Place baking dish containing chicken and marinade in oven, and bake about 35 minutes, or until chicken is no longer pink when tested with a fork. Then broil a few minutes until chicken is golden.

Stuffed Chicken Scallops

Serves 4

Ingredients

- 675g scalloped chicken slices
- 15ml olive oil
- 1 red or yellow pepper, cut into strips
- 150g fresh spinach, washed, stalks trimmed
- 375ml grated Swiss cheese
- 50ml freshly grated Parmesan cheese
- ¼ tsp dried thyme
- ¼ tsp dried rosemary
- ¼ tsp dried tarragon
- pinch onion powder
- salt and pepper to taste

Marinade

- 75ml olive oil
- 45ml freshly squeezed orange juice
- 45ml freshly squeezed grapefruit juice
- 2 tbsp freshly squeezed lemon juice
- 2 tbsp freshly squeezed lime juice
- 2 tbsp Dijon mustard
- 2 large cloves garlic, peeled and crushed

In a bowl, whisk together all the marinade ingredients. Add chicken scallops and turn to coat well. Marinate in refrigerator about 1 hour.

Preheat oven to 180°C, 350°F, Gas Mark 4.

In a non-stick skillet, over medium heat, heat olive oil and cook pepper strips 5 minutes. Add spinach, cover and continue cooking 1 to 2 minutes, or until spinach is wilted.

Drain scallops and reserve marinade. Spoon spinach mixture and Swiss cheese onto each scallop, roll, and secure with a toothpick.

On a plate, mix together Parmesan cheese, herbs and onion powder. Dip scallops in marinade, then roll lightly in Parmesan mixture. Season with salt and pepper.

Transfer scallops to a baking dish and bake 20 minutes, or until chicken is no longer pink when tested with a fork.

Chicken Breasts with Lime

Serves 4

Ingredients

- 4 boneless chicken breasts
- 5 garlic cloves – crushed
- 3 limes
- 4 tbsp olive oil
- salt, freshly ground pepper, cayenne

In a bowl, make a marinade of lime juice, olive oil, crushed garlic, salt and pepper. Mix well.

Dust the chicken breasts lightly with cayenne and immerse in the marinade.

Place in the fridge for a few hours, turning from time to time.

Drain the chicken breasts and put them in a roasting tin. Place in a preheated oven 190°C, 375°F, Gas Mark 5 and cook for 30 minutes.

In the meantime, pour the marinade into a pan, bring to the boil and reduce to obtain a thick sauce.

Serve the chicken breasts coated in this sauce.

Broiled Tuna Steaks

Serves 4

Ingredients

- 375ml unsweetened coconut juice
- 50ml freshly squeezed lime juice
- 2 jalapeno or other similar hot peppers, chopped
- 3 large cloves garlic, peeled and crushed
- 2 tsp paprika
- 1 tsp turmeric powder
- ½ tsp onion powder
- ¼ tsp celery salt
- 4 tuna steaks

Mix all ingredients, except tuna steaks, to make a marinade. Add tuna, turning over to coat well. Marinate in refrigerator 5 hours, turning tuna over occasionally.

Preheat broiler.

Transfer tuna to a shallow baking dish, and broil about 4 minutes on each side, or until fish is opaque and flakes easily when tested with a fork.

Poached Fish

Serves 2

Ingredients

- 1.5l water
- 150ml red wine vinegar
- 2 large cloves garlic, peeled and quartered
- 1 celery stick, roughly chopped
- 1 small onion, quartered
- 15ml finely chopped fresh parsley
- 15ml finely chopped fresh chives
- ½ tsp celery salt
- ½ tsp dried Herbes de Provence
- 1 bay leaf
- pinch freshly ground black pepper
- salt and pepper
- 4 fillets of cod or turbot

In a saucepan, bring water to a boil. Add all ingredients except salt, pepper and fish, cover, and simmer 30 minutes.

Strain the stock through a fine-mesh sieve, and return to saucepan. Bring back to a boil, then turn heat down. Season fish fillets with salt and pepper, and poach in simmering stock 5 minutes, or until fillets are opaque and flake easily when tested with a fork.

Salmon Steaks

Serves 4

Ingredients

- 125ml dry white wine
- 50ml freshly squeezed lemon juice
- 2 tsp olive oil
- 2 large cloves garlic, peeled and crushed
- 15ml finely chopped fresh parsley
- ½ tsp dried tarragon
- salt and pepper to taste
- 4 salmon steaks

In a large bowl, mix all ingredients except salmon. Add salmon steaks, turning over to coat well. Marinate in refrigerator about 1 hour.

Preheat broiler.

Arrange salmon steaks in an ovenproof dish, and broil about 5 minutes on each side, or until fish is opaque and flakes easily when tested with a fork.

Salmon Tidbits

Serves 2

Ingredients

- 225g cooked salmon
- 50ml chopped celery
- 2 green onions, finely sliced
- 1 large egg, beaten
- 15ml freshly grated Romano cheese
- 15ml oat bran
- 45ml finely chopped fresh parsley
- 15ml finely chopped fresh dill
- ¼ tsp celery salt
- freshly ground black pepper to taste
- 15ml olive oil

In a large bowl, combine cooked salmon, celery, onions, egg, cheese, bran and seasonings. Shape into 12 portions. In a large non-stick skillet, over medium heat, heat olive oil, and cook salmon portions 3 to 4 minutes on either side, or until hot and golden.

Variation: Use tuna instead of salmon.

Seafood Brochettes

Serves 4

Ingredients

- 12 large shrimp, shelled and deveined
- 12 large scallops
- 12 small onions, peeled
- 12 cherry tomatoes
- 1 green pepper, cut into large pieces

Marinade

- 175ml olive oil
- 2 tbsp freshly squeezed lemon juice
- 15ml freshly squeezed lime juice
- 1 large clove garlic, peeled and crushed
- salt and pepper to taste
- 2 tbsp grated fresh ginger
- 15ml finely chopped fresh dill

In a bowl, mix marinade ingredients, reserving a quarter for basting. Put shrimp and scallops in marinade and refrigerate about 45 minutes.

Boil onions in lightly salted water until tender.

Preheat oven to 230°C, 450°F, Gas Mark 8.

Thread marinated shrimp and scallops onto metal skewers, alternating with vegetables. Baste onions, tomatoes and pepper with rest of marinade. Bake about 10 minutes, turning over and basting midway through cooking.

Sole en Papillote

Serves 4

Ingredients

- 2 tbsp olive oil
- 1 small red onion, finely chopped
- ½ yellow pepper, cut into strips
- 2 tbsp pesto sauce
- 125ml dry white wine
- 4 medium ripe tomatoes, peeled and roughly chopped
- 8 black olives, pitted and thinly sliced
- 1 tbsp capers
- 1 small clove garlic, peeled and crushed
- salt and freshly ground pepper to taste
- 4 sole fillets
- 2 tbsp freshly squeezed lime juice

In a skillet, over medium heat, heat olive oil, add onion, pepper and pesto, and cook 5 minutes. Add wine and bring to boil. Reduce heat and simmer 3 to 4 minutes or until liquid has evaporated. Add tomatoes, olives and capers, and continue cooking 5 minutes more or until sauce has thickened. Season with salt and pepper.

Preheat oven to 220°C, 425°F, Gas Mark 7. Wipe fillets with a paper towel, and place each one on a separate sheet of aluminium foil about 15 inches (40 cm) long. Cover with sauce and sprinkle lime juice over. Fold aluminium foil over fillets, turn edges in and pinch to seal.

Bake about 15 minutes, or until fish is opaque and flakes easily when tested with a fork. *Note: To peel tomatoes, plunge into boiling water 30 seconds; skin will slide off easily.*

Spicy Shrimp with Ginger

Serves 3 to 4

Ingredients

- 450g large fresh shrimp, shelled and deveined
- ½ tsp paprika
- ½ tsp Cajun seasoning
- ¼ tsp chilli powder
- ⅛ tsp cayenne pepper
- pinch onion powder
- 15ml olive oil
- 1 large clove garlic, peeled and crushed
- 15ml grated fresh ginger
- juice of 1 fresh lime

In a bowl, combine seasonings. Add shrimp and stir to coat.

In a skillet, over medium-high heat, heat oil and cook shrimp 2 minutes. Add garlic and ginger. Season with salt and pepper; and add lime juice. Cook 1 to 2 minutes more, or until shrimp turn pink.

Trout Surprise

Serves 4

Ingredients

- 125ml sour cream
- 50ml plain yoghurt
- 1 tbsp finely chopped red onion
- 1 tbsp finely chopped fresh chives
- 1 tsp finely chopped fresh dill
- olive oil
- 4 trout fillets
- freshly ground black pepper to taste

Preheat oven to 220°C, 425 °F, Gas Mark 7.

In a mixing bowl, combine sour cream, yoghurt, onion and herbs.

Arrange fillets in a lightly oiled ovenproof dish, season with pepper and cover with sour cream sauce.

Bake uncovered 12 minutes. Cover with aluminium foil and bake 5 minutes more, or until fish is opaque and flakes easily when tested with a fork.

Lemon and Apple Creams

Serves 4

Ingredients

- 4 egg yolks
- 1 complete egg
- 3 tbsp fructose
- 2 Golden Delicious apples (peeled), 400g
- 1½ lemons

Beat the egg and the egg yolks together with the fructose. Add the zest of a lemon and the strained juice of 1 lemon.

Grate the apples finely and add to the mixture. Pour into 4 buttered ramekins and cook in a bain-marie at 190 °C, 375 °F, Gas Mark 5 for 30 minutes.

Turn out and serve lukewarm or cold.

Egg Custards

Serves 5

Ingredients

- ½ litre semi-skimmed milk
- 5 egg yolks
- 2 tbsp fructose
- 1 vanilla pod

Heat the milk with the vanilla pod, let it cool slightly and remove the vanilla pod.

Beat the egg yolks vigorously and pour the lukewarm milk over. Add the fructose and pour the mixture into ramekins.

Cook in a bain-marie in a moderate oven (180 °C, 350 °F, Gas Mark 4) for about 30 minutes.

Serve cold in the ramekins.

Floating Islands

Serves 6 to 8

Ingredients

- 1 vanilla pod
- 8 eggs
- 1 litre semi-skimmed milk
- 3 tbsp fructose
- 1 pinch salt

Separate the eggs. Beat the whites until they form stiff peaks, adding a pinch of salt.

Boil the milk with the vanilla pod and half a glass of water. Keep it just simmering. Use a tablespoon to scoop up 'snowballs' of beaten egg white and place on the surface of the milk. Poach them for 1 minute each side, remove and drain on a cloth.

Make an egg custard by beating the egg yolks and adding the lukewarm milk. (Dilute slightly to make the quantity up to 1 litre.) Whisk vigorously. Place on a low heat again to thicken. Sweeten with the fructose at the last minute.

Allow to cool. Serve with the 'snowballs' floating on the custard.

Raspberry Bavarois

Serves 4

Ingredients

- 500g raspberries
- ½ litre milk
- 4 egg yolks
- 3 tbsp fructose
- 3 leaves (1 sachet) gelatine

Bring the milk to the boil. Beat the egg yolks and fructose together in a large bowl. Gradually pour the milk into the bowl, stirring vigorously all the time.

Return to a low heat and cook until the mixture thickens, stirring continuously. Stir in the gelatine; if using leaves, first soften them in cold water and drain.

Blend 200g of the raspberries to a purée and combine this with the custard. Add 50g whole raspberries.

Pour the mixture into ramekins or a charlotte mould and place in the refrigerator for 12 hours to set. Make a raspberry coulis with the remainder of the fruit.

Turn out and serve with the coulis poured over.

Summer Fruits Mousse

Serves 4 to 5

Ingredients

- 250g fromage frais (20% fat)
- 3 egg whites
- 3 tbsp fructose
- 100g raspberries
- 100g small strawberries

Add 1 tbsp of fructose to the egg whites and beat until they form stiff peaks.

Mix the fromage frais with the other 2 tbsp of fructose. Fold in the beaten egg whites gently, to make a mousse.

Wash the fruit and cut into pieces. Fold into the mixture.

Place in a large bowl and chill for a few hours.

Apricot Mousse

Serves 4

Ingredients

- 500g apricots
- 1 lemon
- 2 tbsp fructose
- 2 leaves (two thirds of sachet) gelatine
- 150g fromage frais (20% fat)
- 100g low-fat cream

Blanch the apricots in boiling water for 1 minute. Drain, skin and cut in half to remove the stone.

Blend to a purée and add the lemon juice and the fructose. If using gelatine leaves, soften in cold water and drain. Melt the gelatine in 2 tbsp water in a bain-marie and immediately combine with the apricot purée.

Whip the fromage frais and add to the mixture, combining thoroughly.

Pour the mousse into ramekins and set in the refrigerator for 3 hours.

Serve well chilled.

Mango Sorbet

Serves 4

Ingredients

- 2 ripe mangoes (providing 450g flesh)
- 1 small tin of condensed, unsweetened, semi-skimmed milk
- 2 tbsp lemon juice
- few drops vanilla essence
- 2 tbsp fructose

Peel and stone the mangoes and chop the flesh into small pieces.

Blend with the condensed milk, the lemon juice, vanilla essence and fructose (the consistency should be light and frothy).

Place the mousse in the freezer for about 3 hours. Use a scoop to serve, as if it were ice-cream.

Recommendation: Use a sorbet-maker for best results.

Chocolate Soufflé

Serves 6

Ingredients

- 200g dark chocolate with 70% minimum cocoa solids
- 5 eggs
- 40ml milk
- 25g single cream
- few drops lemon juice

Preheat the oven to 190°C, 375°F, Gas Mark 5. Break the chocolate into pieces and melt in a bain-marie. Away from the heat, add the milk, cream, and egg yolks, stirring continuously with a whisk.

Add the lemon juice to the egg whites and beat until they form stiff peaks. Fold gently into the chocolate mixture, a little at a time.

Butter a 17cm soufflé mould and pour the mixture into it. Cook in the oven, turned down to the lowest setting, for 20 minutes.

Serve immediately so that the soufflé does not collapse.

Coconut Custard with Berries

Serves 6

Ingredients

- 2 large whole eggs
- 4 large egg yolks
- 50ml fructose
- ¼ tsp salt
- ¼ tsp pure vanilla extract
- 500ml milk
- 45ml unsweetened grated coconut
- 45ml chopped walnuts (optional)
- berries (raspberries, strawberries, blackberries)

Preheat oven to 150°C, 300°F, Gas Mark 2. In a mixing bowl, beat whole eggs, egg yolks, fructose, salt and vanilla extract. In a saucepan, bring milk to barely simmering, and beat in egg mixture.

Pour into 6 individual ramekins; place into a shallow pan of water, and bake 1 hour.

Unmould each ramekin onto a plate, sprinkle coconut and nuts over, and serve with whole berries, or a purée of berries.

Frozen Chocolate Yoghurt

Serves 4

Ingredients

- 100g unsweetened chocolate, containing at least 70% chocolate liquor or cocoa
- 375ml plain yoghurt
- 50ml fructose
- 1 large egg white

Break chocolate into pieces, and melt in a double boiler (or bain-marie) with 1 tbsp water, stirring with a spatula.

In a bowl, beat yoghurt with fructose for 1 minute. Gradually add melted chocolate, beating constantly, until well blended. Spread mixture in a large dish and freeze at least 8 hours.

Using a knife, cut frozen mixture into pieces. Transfer to food processor and process just until pieces are smaller. Add egg white, and process until mixture is creamy.

Serve immediately.

Variation: Add 2 to 3 tbsp ground almonds or hazelnuts to yoghurt-chocolate mixture before freezing.

Raspberry Bavarian Cream

Serves 8

Ingredients

- 500ml raspberries, fresh or frozen and defrosted
- 2 tbsp unsweetened gelatine powder
- 125ml cold water
- 50ml boiling water
- 75ml fructose
- 15ml freshly squeezed lime juice
- 1 tsp pure vanilla extract
- 2 large egg whites
- 250ml whipping cream, whipped
- fresh mint leaves and whole raspberries for garnish

In a food processor or blender, purée raspberries, and set aside.

In a bowl, sprinkle gelatine over cold water and let stand 5 minutes. Add boiling water, stirring until gelatine is dissolved. Add raspberry purée, half the fructose, lime juice and vanilla extract. Stir well, and refrigerate (stirring occasionally) about 20 minutes or until mixture has thickened.

In a separate bowl, beat egg whites, add remaining fructose and continue beating until soft peaks have formed. Gently fold egg whites into raspberry mixture, then fold in cream.

Pour into individual ramekins, and refrigerate at least 3 hours, until set. Unmould Bavarian creams onto a serving dish, and garnish with mint leaves and raspberries.

Raspberry Snow

Serves 4

Ingredients

- 500ml raspberries, fresh or frozen and thawed
- 50ml fructose
- 250ml plain yoghurt
- 50ml low-fat sour cream
- ¼ tsp freshly grated orange zest
- ¼ tsp pure vanilla extract
- fresh mint leaves for garnish

In a mixing bowl, combine raspberries and fructose. Let stand 20 minutes, stirring occasionally.

In another bowl, combine yoghurt, sour cream, orange zest and vanilla extract.

Divide a third of the raspberry mixture into 4 sorbet glasses; to each add 2 tbsp yoghurt mixture. Repeat procedure with a layer of raspberry mixture, and a layer of yoghurt mixture.

Top with remaining raspberry mixture, and finish with 1 tbsp of yoghurt mixture. Garnish with mint leaves and serve.

Strawberry Coulis

Makes 300ml

Ingredients

- 500ml strawberries, fresh or frozen and defrosted
- 1-2 tbsp fructose
- 1 tsp freshly squeezed lime juice

In a blender or food processor, purée strawberries. Transfer purée to a small saucepan, add fructose and lime juice, and cook over low heat 10 minutes, stirring occasionally.

Serve hot or at room temperature.

Variation: Use raspberries or kiwi fruit instead of strawberries.

Serving tip: Delicious served with custard or crème caramel.

Grilled Pear Zabaglione

Serves 4

Ingredients

- 8 good pears
- 100g fructose
- 5 egg yolks
- juice of 1 orange
- 1 tsp vanilla extract
- 1 tbsp rum
- mint leaves

Peel the pears, quarter and remove the cores. Slice each quarter into two.

Arrange the pear slices on the bottom of an ovenware dish lightly brushed with oil. Sprinkle 25g fructose over the top. Place under the grill for 5 to 10 minutes, to allow the pears to brown lightly without burning. Reserve.

To make the sabayon, whisk the egg yolks and fructose together until they begin to turn slightly white and creamy. Add the orange juice, vanilla, rum and cooking juice from the pears.

Cook gently in a bain-marie, beating constantly, until the cream thickens slightly.

Arrange the pear slices on serving plates. Pour the cream over the top and decorate with a mint leaf.